Travel Health Nursing
1st edition

Scope and Standards of Practice

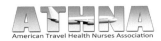

American Travel Health Nurses Association

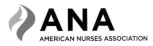

AMERICAN NURSES ASSOCIATION

American Nurses Association
Silver Spring, Maryland 2021

The American Travel Health Nurses Association (ATHNA) and the American Nurses Association (ANA) are national professional associations. This joint ATHNA and ANA publication—*Travel Health Nursing: Scope and Standards of Practice*—reflects the position of ATHNA regarding the specialty practice of travel health nursing and should be reviewed in conjunction with state board of nursing regulations. State law rules and regulations govern the practice of nursing, while *Travel Health Nursing: Scope and Standards of Practice* guides travel health registered nurses in the application of their professional skills and responsibilities.

About the American Travel Health Nurses Association

The American Travel Health Nurses Association (ATHNA) is the professional association of travel health nurses in the United States. ATHNA defines the scope and sets standards for the specialty, advocates for quality health and safety for all travelers and the communities they impact worldwide, promotes the professional development of its members, and collaborates with local, national, and international partners to advance the specialty through evidence-based practice, ethical conduct, education, and research.

American Travel Health Nurses Association
3E Evergreen Rd #1024
New City, NY 10956

About the American Nurses Association

The American Nurses Association (ANA) is the only full-service professional organization representing the interests of the nation's 4.2 million registered nurses through its constituent/state nurses associations and its organizational affiliates. The ANA advances the nursing profession by fostering high standards of nursing practice, promoting the rights of nurses in the workplace, projecting a positive and realistic view of nursing, and by lobbying the Congress and regulatory agencies on healthcare issues affecting nurses and the public.

American Nurses Association
8515 Georgia Avenue, Suite 400
Silver Spring, MD 20910

ISBN-
Print: 978-1-947800-81-6
ePDF 978-1-947800-82-3
ePUB 978-1-947800-83-0
Mobi: 978-1-947800-84-7
SAN: 851-3481

Contents

Contributors

The American Travel Health Nurses Association (ATHNA) Scope and Standards Task Force

Sue Ann McDevitt, BSN, RN, FISTM, FATHNA, AFTM, RCPS (Glasg)

Julie Richards, MS, MSN, WHNP-BC, FNP-BC, FATHNA

Mette Riis, MSW, BSN, RN

Elaine Rosenblatt, MSN, FNP-BC, FATHNA

Gail Rosselot, MS, MPH, APRN-BC, FAANP, FISTM, FATHNA, FFTM, RCPS (Glasg)—Chair

Candace Sandal, DNP, APRN-BC, FAAOHN

Sandy Weinberg, MA, BSN, RN, FATHNA

ANA Staff

Carol J. Bickford, PhD, RN-BC, CPHIMS, FHIMSS, FAAN—Content editor

Erin E. Walpole, BA, PMP—Project editor

ANA Committee on Nursing Practice Standards

Nena M. Bonuel, PhD, RN, CCRN-K, APRN-BC

Patricia Bowe, DNP, MS, RN

Danette Culver, MSN, APRN, ACNS-BC, CCRN

Elizabeth O. Dietz, EdD, RN, CS-NP, Alternate

Kirk Koyama, MSN, RN, CNS, PHN, Co-Chair

Tonette McAndrew, MPA, RN

Stacy McNall, MSN, RN, IBCLC

Verna Sitzer, PhD, RN, CNS

Mona Pearl Treyball, PhD, RN, CNS, CCRN-K, FAAN

Jordan Wilson, BSN, RN, Alternate

Introduction

Scope and Standards of Travel Health Nursing

The American Travel Health Nurses Association (ATHNA) is the specialty nursing organization for travel health nurses in the United States. ATHNA establishes, maintains, and promotes the standards for professional travel health nursing practice.

Definitions

Travel health nursing is the specialized nursing practice that advances the well-being of all travelers in all phases/stages of travel and in all settings. This specialty focuses on the health and safety of travelers through continuous surveillance and assessment of the multiple determinants of health with the intent to promote health and wellness; and prevent disease, disability, and premature death. Travel health nursing is a highly complex nursing specialty that draws on knowledge from nursing, pharmacology, epidemiology, tropical medicine, primary care, and behavioral psychology to provide evidence-based interventions that ensure the health and safety of travelers and the communities they impact.

Travel health nursing professionals represent the myriad of specially educated and trained registered nurses, advanced practice registered nurses, and graduate-level prepared travel health nurses who exercise the expert nursing process skills of assessing patients, analyzing subjective and objective data pertinent to travel, educating patients about travel-related health risks and safety concerns, as well as teaching health promotion and illness avoidance. The methods of this specialty are evidence-based and in accordance with professional and ethical standards. Travel health nurses practice within the scope of their state nurse practice acts and the standards of the specialty. They function as direct care providers and consultants to businesses, organizations, and the traveling public. Travel health nurses are researchers, faculty members, and nursing leaders. Many are entrepreneurs, serving as owners and operators of their own travel health centers.

The American Nurses Association (ANA) document, *Nursing: Scope and Standards of Practice, 3rd Edition* (ANA, 2015b) defines the practice of professional nursing in the United States. It is the foundation for this publication ATHNA's and ANA's, *Travel Health Nursing: Scope and Standards of Practice, 1st Edition,* (2021), which describes the specialty of travel health nursing. This scope of practice statement provides a comprehensive description of travel health nursing: the what, when, where, who, how, and why of the specialty practice. The standards guide the practice of travel health nurses and the quality nursing care of travelers. The standards serve to maintain safe and competent clinical and administrative practice as travel health nursing roles and responsibilities evolve.

Travel health nursing is a dynamic and evolving specialty, and this publication updates ATHNA's *Travel Health Nursing: Scope and Standards of Practice* II (self-published 2014). It includes an expanded scope of practice statement and 17 standards with competencies for the professional practice of travel health nursing in an increasingly "complex global healthcare environment" (Hill 2016). The standards for travel health nursing are intentionally general and broad to encompass the expanding responsibilities of travel health nurses. The accompanying competencies explain how the standards apply to general travel health nursing practice and, therefore, may be modified for a specific travel health nursing population or setting.

The purpose of this publication is to:

1. Provide concrete information for travel health nurses, other health professionals, and the public about what constitutes travel health nursing practice provided by registered nurses, advance practice registered nurses and graduate-level prepared travel health nurses.

2. Promote and guide the delivery of pre- and post-travel quality nursing care for individuals, families, and groups in diverse outpatient settings (e.g., policies, procedures, and competencies).

3. Raise standards of practice and achieve greater uniformity in the provision of travel health nursing services to better protect travelers.

4. Facilitate the development and dissemination of professional nursing knowledge in travel health in the undergraduate, graduate, and continuing education (CE) environments.

5. Serve as a resource to travel health nurses and their employers for job descriptions, orientation manuals, ongoing training, and professional promotion.

6. Facilitate the evaluation of professional travel health nursing performance as evidenced in performance appraisals, peer reviews, and reflective practice.

7. Serve as a reference for the scope and performance standards of travel health nursing for use by governments and the legal system.

8. Promote participation in travel health nursing research and evidence-based practice.

9. Guide performance improvement initiatives in clinical and organizational environments.

10. Guide and promote ethical practice.

11. Serve as a vehicle to advance the specialty of travel health nursing and improve health outcomes for travelers and the communities to which they travel and return.

History of Travel Health Nursing Standards

The concept that specific travel health nursing standards were needed started sometime in the 1990s. Nurses in the United States had been directed by employers to provide care to travelers for more than 10 years. All too often, however, nurses were asked to provide pre-travel services based solely on their experience of providing allergy injections or routine immunizations; nurses were rarely afforded any specialized education or training to address the varied health issues related to travel. Indeed, it was not uncommon for a nurse working in a corporate or college health setting to be expected to prepare international travelers in a brief encounter that was simply added to the clinic schedule with little or no prior notice. Safety and security information for the destination were not routinely addressed. The many needs of travelers beyond immunization services were rarely recognized.

The necessity for nursing standards was also raised as a frequent topic for discussion whenever travel health nurses around the country engaged in networking and professional development. Travel health nurses voiced valid concerns about inconsistencies in the delivery of pre- and post-travel nursing care; they also raised questions about patient safety, undue influence of pharmaceutical representatives, potential conflicts of interest in for-profit settings, and the lack of training opportunities in travel health.

At about the same time, travel health nurses at the Royal College of Nursing (RCN) in the United Kingdom started to develop a set of competencies for travel health nurses in their country; they too, saw the need for travelers to receive quality services that went beyond the delivery of vaccinations. U.S. nurses learned about the RCN initiative at international conferences and then established communications with nursing principals that included Jane Chiodini and Sandra Grieves. Additionally, nurses learned about the travel health course offered by the Faculty of Travel Medicine at the Royal College of Physicians and Surgeons of Glasgow. Subsequently, U.S. travel health nurses learned of additional professional efforts in the Netherlands.

In 2004, when ATHNA was incorporated, the initial goal was to document the scope and standards of travel health nursing. This effort was seen as a fundamental and necessary step to both define the specialty and help ensure safe and consistent pre- and post-travel nursing care for travelers. That first self-published version was modeled on the ANA *Nursing: Scope and Standards of Practice* with additional attention paid to the published work of travel health nurses in the United Kingdom and the Netherlands, and publications of the Centers for Disease Control and Prevention (CDC), the World Health Organization (WHO), the Infectious Disease Society of America (IDSA), and the International Society of Travel Medicine (ISTM).

Starting in 2012, ATHNA initiated a working group to explore formal recognition of travel health nursing as a specialty. Toward that goal, in 2014, ATHNA revised its *Travel Health Nursing: Scope and Standards of Practice* I (self-published 2004), again using the model of the latest ANA scope and standards edition. That second edition of ATHNA's *Travel Health Nursing: Scope and Standards of Practice,* II (self-published 2014) included competencies for each of the standards and descriptions of the various professional nursing roles. In 2017, ATHNA made ANA recognition of travel health nursing as an official nursing specialty its number one organizational priority. As part of that effort, this edition of the *Travel Health Nursing: Scope and Standards of Practice, 1st Edition (2021)* was developed in accordance with the 2015 requirements of ANA. This latest edition includes an expanded scope of practice statement to more fully document the travel health nursing specialty as well as expanded competencies. In addition, ATHNA created an application of the provisions of *ANA's Code of Ethics for Nurses with Interpretive Statements* for travel health nurses, *Application of Code of Ethics Provisions by Travel Health Nurses.*

Scope of Travel Health Nursing: The What, When, Where, Who, How, and Why

The scope of a nursing specialty defines the specialty and describes what it involves, where it is practiced, who provides the care, and the how and why of specialty practice.

Scope of Travel Health Nursing: The WHAT

As previously mentioned, travel health nursing focuses on the health and safety of all travelers through continuous surveillance and assessment of the multiple determinants of health with the intent to promote health and wellness; and prevent disease, disability, and premature death. It is a highly complex nursing specialty that draws on knowledge from nursing, pharmacology, epidemiology, tropical medicine, primary care and behavioral psychology to provide evidence-based interventions that contribute to the health and safety of domestic and international travelers and the communities they impact.

Objectives of Travel Health Nursing

- The travel health nurse uses the nursing process to promote the health and safety of travelers, the destinations to which they travel, and the communities to which they return.

- The travel health nurse assesses subjective and objective data obtained from the patient, as well as authoritative national and international travel health resources to structure an outpatient encounter focusing on illness prevention and health promotion, including safety and security information for the traveler. The goal is to prepare travelers to achieve a healthy and safe trip that meets their personal goals.

- The travel health nurse individualizes patient care in the context of caring, compassion, and sensitivity to multiple traveler and trip factors: age, gender, ethnicity, culture, health status, previous travel history, reason for travel, finances, length of trip, planned events during the trip, and time before departure.

- The travel health nurse customizes patient care utilizing the most up-to-date national and international global health and safety risk data. Travel risks may include vaccine-preventable and non-vaccine-preventable infectious diseases, seasonal, climate, and altitude risks, food- and water-borne illnesses, transportation accidents, activity risks (e.g., fresh water swimming, spelunking, ocean sports, mountaineering, etc.), sexually transmitted infections (STIs), social unrest, crime, disease outbreaks, and access to, and quality of, medical and safety services. The travel health nurse incorporates the teach-back method with the traveler to verbalize how these risks are to be managed while abroad in order to evaluate how well the education was received.

- The travel health nurse performs a comprehensive health and safety risk assessment customized to the traveler and itinerary, utilizing appropriate reliable resources (CDC, WHO, etc.) to develop and implement an evidence-based nursing plan of risk reduction using pharmaceutical and nonpharmaceutical interventions, and evaluates outcomes for travelers, their destination(s), and their home community.

- The travel health nurse triages the ill or injured post-travel patient with special attention to the serious, treatable, and transmissible. If a transmissible illness is identified, the travel health nurse will notify the proper authorities and take action to protect the local community and traveler as indicated.

- The travel health nurse participates in ongoing education, research, and advocacy to implement/translate learning to actions in order to achieve continuous improvements in the 1) pre- and post-travel care of travelers, 2) global coordination and implementation of health and safety measures that benefit all populations, and 3) advancement of the practice of travel health nursing.

Travel Health Nursing Encounters

Nurses in this specialty provide services in three different clinical encounters: pre-travel, during travel ("in-transit"), and post-travel. In addition, travel health nurses can provide a variety of administrative and educational nursing services, such as seminars for healthcare personnel and groups of travelers, and consultations to organizations and providers who have questions about a challenging travel encounter.

Pre-Travel Encounters

Travel health nurses provide direct nursing care in a variety of outpatient settings and by tele-health and electronic messaging. Travel health nurses provide pre-travel care visits to individuals, families, and groups. The clinical encounter is episodic and time-limited. While a single visit is common, multiple visits for a particular trip or multiple itineraries may be required either to complete the assessment, and/or an immunization series or for extended health counseling. Additionally, travel health nurses provide expert consultation encounters to promote travel-related health and safety of groups and organizations. Moreover, they are indispensable speakers to audiences new to the idea of international travel, as the expertise of travel health nurses is freely shared regarding the benefits of seeing our nation and the world, as well as current requirements and recommendations for vaccine-preventable diseases with practical advice regarding self-care in order to optimize health and safety while on a journey.

Most travelers initiate the travel health nursing clinical encounter as they prepare for international or domestic travel; alternatively, some travelers are directed to travel health nursing care by employers, school authorities, tour managers, the military, and others. The assessment phase of the encounter encompasses a largely self-reported traveler health history. Next, health and safety risks for a given itinerary (destination and activity risks) are identified using sophisticated internet-based search engines. At the heart of the assessment is a complex risk analysis, considering both the likelihood as well as the consequences of specific health and safety occurrences. Risk factors related to the traveler include age, possibility of pregnancy, allergies, chronic illness, unstable medical and psychiatric conditions, previous immunizations, previous travel-related illnesses and medications. Additional risks include: risk-taking tendencies as they relate to sexual behavior, drug use and extreme sports, travel health insurance coverage, travel motivation, concerns, attitudes, country restrictions, and status as an immigrant or refugee or "Visiting Friends and Relatives" (VFR) traveler. Risk factors related to the trip include destination(s), departure dates, specific order of countries to be visited, duration in each country (especially greater than one month), season, climate, and altitude at destinations, type of accommodations, trip purpose, specific activities, and modes of transportation.

International and domestic travel expands every year in terms of numbers, destinations, and reasons for travel. Increasingly, travel health nurses are called upon to provide individualized care to travelers who are making trips that go beyond typical vacation, employee, and VFR travel. Pre-travel encounters include care for unaccompanied minors, expats, flexpats, medical and dental tourists, romance tourists, ecotourists, students (school and college), researchers, missioners, babymooners, voluntourists, military and emergency responders. They also include care for pilgrims, specialty tourists: food, spa, adventure, history, LGBTQ+, solo, and single parent, space traveler, green traveler, cruise traveler, war zone traveler, bucket list travelers, disaster response workers and volunteers, sex tourists, persons adopting internationally, intergenerational tourists, remote travelers, immigrants, and refugees. As more travelers seek medical or dental care internationally, the expectation that a traveler is "in good health" is no longer valid. To add to this concern are travelers with special needs and who require assistive devices, are oxygen dependent, have a companion animal, or need syringes or other specialized equipment and supplies to manage illnesses, such as diabetes, psoriatic arthritis, or bleeding disorders.

Travel health nurses can also expect to prepare travelers with a wide range of physical and mental health issues that can include chronic physical illness (e.g., COPD, CHF, DM, RA, severe allergies, severe motion sickness, asplenia) and mild to severe psychological conditions (e.g., OCD, ADHD, panic attacks, depression, bipolar disorder, eating disorders, addictions, flying phobias). Travel health nurses will also prepare individuals who are pregnant or trying to conceive, post-surgical patients, persons with immunosuppressive conditions and therapies, travelers with new diagnoses currently being investigated, conditions requiring the use of medications either not available internationally or outlawed at the destination, and medical or dental issues that will be addressed with services in another country.

During the implementation phase of the encounter, the travel health nurse provides pharmaceutical interventions (immunizations, medications within state scope of nursing practice guidelines) and nonpharmaceutical interventions (health counseling, coordination of care with other health providers, referrals for additional evaluation, and care and guidance for post-trip health management). A typical visit may include the administration of routine vaccinations (including any necessary catch-up doses or boosters) and vaccines that are recommended or required for travel as well as customized counseling to prevent traveler's diarrhea, vector-borne infections that include malaria, Aedes illnesses (e.g., dengue, Zika, yellow fever), and rabies, STIs, motor vehicle accidents, airline hazards (e.g., deep vein thrombosis [DVT], jet lag, respiratory infections), climate hazards, and fresh water-related illnesses.

Many travelers will require a review of their routine medications, as well as guidance for the use of drugs indicated for certain travel-related risks (altitude illness, traveler's diarrhea, malaria) and recommendations for the assembly of a personalized travel medical kit. Travelers with pre-existing conditions will receive self-care management counseling and education about medical services and access abroad. Travel health nurses will document the encounter in the health record and also complete any necessary medical documents required by a government (e.g. visa application), or a tour company, employer, camp, school, or college. They will issue the *International Certificate of Vaccination or Prophylaxis* (ICVP) card, if a required vaccine is administered, provide a waiver if yellow fever vaccine is medically contraindicated, and provide medical letters that travelers may need or want to carry on the trip (e.g., explaining a chronic condition or the use of an injectable medication). The travel health nurse may also assist in the translation of these documents into the primary language of the destination.

Every traveler during the pre-travel encounter receives guidance about post-travel care that may include a timeline for additional vaccine doses or boosters, urgent follow-up for febrile illness, the need to complete a malaria medication schedule, post-trip behaviors after travel to Zika regions (pregnancy avoidance, use of repellents), and recognition of signs and symptoms that warrant medical attention upon return. Travelers are also reminded that they could return home with infections that necessitate rapid attention to prevent community spread. Time spent in the pre-travel encounter is valuable for assessing adverse vaccine reactions and providing instantaneous management of same. The encounter also offers the traveler role play and teach-back opportunities of common health issues encountered during travel to confirm traveler knowledge of counseling content and correct responses. As travelers with more complex needs are cared for during the pre-travel encounter, the scope and complexity of travel health nursing practice has broadened and increased. This can be especially true of travelers who are older, pregnant, foreign-borne, or with comorbidities related to chronic disease and disability.

Travel health nurses with prescriptive authority will also prescribe travel medications during the pre-travel encounter that may include, but are not limited to, therapies for altitude illness, malaria, traveler's diarrhea, skin infections, respiratory infections, chronic illnesses such as asthma or diabetes, severe allergic reactions, contraception, UTIs, and musculoskeletal injuries.

In-Transit Encounters

With advances in communication technology, travel health nurses may be called upon to offer patient counseling, arrange for referrals, or order prescriptions for travelers in transit almost anywhere in the world. For example, patients may call to say that their malaria medication is causing problematic side effects, and they want a referral to a destination clinic for a replacement drug. Assistance with evacuation from Israel for a traveler with an acute case of "Jerusalem Syndrome" (psychotic episode with associated religious obsessions or delusions) would be another example. In addition to these at-a-distance contacts, travel health nurses can travel with a group and serve as the designated, on-site health care provider. As a result of in-transit encounters and on-the-scene travel encounters, the travel health nurse may recommend changes to site pre-travel and post-travel policies and procedures, as well as suggestions for travel medical kits and staff training.

Post-Travel Encounters

In post-travel encounters, travel health nurses will, in accordance with the parameters of their state nursing scope of practice and institutional policies, provide triage, health evaluation, medical and nursing diagnosis, and management of health problems encountered during a journey. These problems may include trauma, routine illness, infections, and tropical or more exotic emerging diseases. The travel health nurse providing post-travel care focuses on the infectious versus the non-infectious, and proceeds to evaluate and manage the serious, treatable, and transmissible based on his or her level of training and practice in accordance with site protocols, referring as appropriate. The goal is to treat the patient, while preventing transmission to others and reporting to institutional and public health authorities as appropriate.

During the assessment phase of a post-travel encounter, the travel health nurse must answer some initial critical questions: Is there a risk to self? Is there a risk to others? How much time is available? The process is quite complicated as many illnesses present in a similar fashion with flu-like symptoms.

Life-threatening illnesses can initially appear benign, and the differential diagnosis can be quite large. Since an illness like *Plasmodium falciparum* malaria can be fatal very quickly, timely intervention is critical.

The first step is to determine what personal protective equipment is needed and if isolation is necessary. A thorough history is essential. The travel health nurse will ask the traveler about signs and symptoms of illness, as well as dates of onset, and then collect information on a number of variables that can contribute to trip-related illness, including, but not limited to, all geographic destinations and associated dates, routine and travel immunizations, seasonal and cultural factors, food, water, and insect precautions, accommodations, ectoparasites, modes of travel, local contacts, compliance with personal protective measures (PPM) and medications. Additional trip variables include any animal contacts, freshwater exposure, medical or dental care abroad, trip purpose and activities, number of new sexual partners, consumption of reef fish, unpasteurized dairy products or bush meat, and outbreaks. The travel health nurse will make the necessary referrals for further evaluation. If the ill traveler is a member of a group or organization, the travel health nurse will take additional actions to provide surveillance and evaluate other members of the group as warranted. In the event of communicable disease risk, the travel health nurse will take measures to ensure the safety of other patients and staff and notify the appropriate public health officials immediately.

A travel health Advanced Practice Registered Nurse (APRN) with additional training in post-travel care creates a differential of diagnoses utilizing the traveler's health history, itinerary, and up-to-date information about global health. The travel health nurse will then determine if the patient's complaints are related to travel exposures, unrelated to exposures during the recent trip, or because of past travel or previously forgotten trips. Based on the likelihood of specific illnesses, and taking into account incubation periods and exposure times, the travel health nurse determines any appropriate diagnostic testing.

The travel health APRN implements appropriate treatment measures, including medical therapies and health education. In some circumstances, the travel health nurse recognizes the need to initiate treatment based on history and clinical findings before definitive lab results are available (e.g., malaria or serious rickettsial infections). The travel health nurse refers to other specialists as indicated and provides follow-up as appropriate. Finally, the travel health nurse makes recommendations for future screening for asymptomatic conditions (e.g., schistosomiasis, strongyloides, filariasis, Chagas disease, COVID-19). As a result of this encounter, the travel health nurse may recommend changes to site prevention policies and protocols and staff training.

Administrative and Educational Roles

In addition to clinical encounters, travel health nurses are often called upon to provide consultation services, utilizing their assessment, risk reduction, and analytical skills to advise groups and organizations pre- or post-travel (see Figure 1. Process of Travel Health Nursing). Employers, tour companies, colleges, non-government organizations (NGOs), governments, and other entities (e.g., missioner, adoption, and refugee assistance groups) will seek travel health nursing assessments of potential hazards for a given itinerary and travel health nursing recommendations for primary and secondary prevention measures. For example, the travel health nurse may be asked to recommend appropriate accommodations for a corporate frequent flyer who is morbidly obese or a student with a seizure disorder joining a study abroad group. Travel health nurses may also be asked to identify and assess health care services abroad or confirm the availability of, and sources for, medical equipment (e.g., wheelchairs, oxygen) at destinations. Travel health nurses provide group presentations as part of these consultations and develop relevant policies, standing orders, web content, and CE programs for nurses, physicians, public health officials, and pharmacists and educational materials, such as articles, brochures, and posters for health professionals and the public.

During the pre- and post-travel clinical encounters, travel health nurses actively seek opportunities to improve the care of individuals and family travelers. In an administrative or educational capacity, travel health nurses seek to improve the care of, and outcomes for, travel populations (e.g., employees, students, seniors, immigrants, and refugees). Many travel health clinics in the United States are managed by travel health nurses, utilizing nursing protocols established by travel health nurses. Throughout the United States, travel health nurses engage with local and national stakeholders to maximize the health and safety of travelers and minimize the impact of travel risks on communities here and abroad.

Scope of Travel Health Nursing: The WHEN

Travel health nurses provide care to travelers at any stage of their journey. They most frequently interact with travelers during pre-travel encounters for trip preparation and during post-travel encounters for triage, evaluation, and management of travel-related injury or illness. In addition, individuals, groups, and organizations often engage travel health nurses in the trip planning process to identify and reduce itinerary health and safety risks. During an outbreak or its aftermath, the travel health nurse may also function as part of the response and evaluation team. Travel health nurses routinely design and deliver travel health curricula and educational programs to varied professional groups including nursing, medicine, public health, pharmacy and veterinary

Risk Assessment: Traveler	RISK ASSESSMENT: TRIP
• Experience • Age • Possibility of pregnancy • Chronic illness • Differently abled • Unstable medical/psychiatric condition • Allergies • Risk-taking tendencies-sex, drugs, and extreme sports • Health insurance • Previous immunizations • LGBTQ • Immunocompromised • Travel motivation, concerns, and attitudes • Medications-country restrictions • Those visiting friends and relatives in their countries of origin	• Destination (armed conflict zones, arctic, remote, etc.) • Departure date • Specific order of countries to be visited • Duration in each country (esp. >1 month) • Seasons at destination (monsoons, typhoons, etc.?) • Type of accommodations (camping, hostels, windows/ac, etc.) • Activities (spelunking, diving, extreme sports, high altitude) • Purpose (research, study, missionary, journalism, athlete, adoption, medical tourism) • Modes of transportation • Mass gatherings (Hajj/Umrah/Kumbh Mela, etc.)

RISK ANALYSIS: OUTCOMES VARY WITH SPECIFICS			PRE-TRAVEL PREPARATION

	Consequences Low	Consequences Catastrophic	• Risk assessment
			  • Traveler
			  • Trip
			• Designing a customized plan
			  • Counseling
			  • Immunizations
			  • Medications
			  • Referrals

Likelihood Low	Most chikungunya	Malaria Rabies Typhoid fever Hemorrhagic Dengue	
Likelihood High	Traveler's Diarrhea Most dengue Most zika	Malaria Rabies Typhoid fever	

POST-TRAVEL CARE	RELIABLE RESOURCES
• Establish differential diagnosis • Perform appropriate diagnostic tests • Recommend appropriate treatments and follow-up • Notify any appropriate public health officials as indicated	• Centers for Disease Control • Subscription services such as Travax, TravelCare • ProMED-mail • Immunization Action Coalition • International Association for Medical Assistance to Travelers • Gideon Database • World Health Organization

Figure 1. Process of Travel Health Nursing.

medicine, as well as lay audiences. At any time, travel health nurses may be called upon by clinics, institutions, communities, and governments to develop policies and procedures that promote the health and safety of travelers and their destinations. Travel health nurses actively participate in clinical services that receive and care for immigrants and refugees as well. Travel health nurses provide tele-health services to travelers in transit and also serve as accompanying healthcare providers on group trips, such as treks and safaris. Travel health nurses are actively involved in travel health research and writing for peer and lay publications on diverse travel-related health topics (e.g., repellent choices, Zika, transporting medications abroad). They manage clinical travel health services and serve in leadership roles in professional organizations, academic settings, and governmental groups. The scope of travel health nursing encompasses the full range of roles, functions, responsibilities, and activities the travel health nurse has the authority to perform when the patient is a traveler or a health or safety issue involves travel to any destination, domestic or international. Travel health nursing is the specialized nursing practice that advances the well-being of travelers to all destinations, in all phases/stages of travel, and in all settings.

Scope of Travel Health Nursing: The WHERE
Travel Health Nursing Practice Sites

Travel health nurses provide clinical services to individuals, families, and groups in a variety of outpatient settings in the United States and abroad including:

- Hospital outpatient clinics
- Emergency rooms
- Group multispecialty practices
- Solo practices: internal medicine, family practice, pediatrics, ob-gyn, infectious disease
- Nurse-owned or managed practices
- Travel health clinics
- Tele-health call centers
- Pharmacies
- School health centers
- College health centers
- Occupational health units
- Public health departments

- Military bases
- Urgent care centers
- Visiting Nurse Associations
- Government offices (CIA, FBI, U.S. embassies, etc.)

Consumers can find travel health nurses for clinical services in a number of different ways. Corporate and government employees often find them at worksite clinics. Students, faculty, administration, and staff at colleges and universities locate their services at their institutions. County and public health organizations maintain listings of travel health nursing services available to the public. The VNA and the military offer travel health nursing services. CDC publishes a list of all travel health clinics that offer the yellow fever vaccine in the United States. HealthMap Vaccine Finder and the CDC Flu Vaccine Finder are two websites that direct travelers to travel health nursing resources in or near their zip code. Both the International Society of Travel Medicine (ISTM) and the International Association for Medical Assistance to Travellers (IAMAT) list travel health clinics around the world by country. In addition to these listings, other health professionals in a community, such as primary care providers and specialists, often refer their patients to travel health nurses for pre- and post-travel care.

In addition to the delivery of direct patient care services, travel health nurses function as consultants to businesses, religious and humanitarian organizations, educational institutions, and NGOs. They serve as faculty members at nursing, medicine, and public health schools as well as regional, national, and international professional conferences. They are researchers and nursing leaders, and some are entrepreneurs, serving as owners and operators of their own travel health centers.

Scope of Travel Health Nursing: The WHO
Professional Nursing Designations

Travel health nurses are licensed at all levels of nursing. While as yet there is no specific graduate degree in the specialty, many travel health nurses hold a variety of graduate degrees including nursing, public health, health education, and health administration (MS, MSN, MPH, MBA, PhD, and DNP). Travel health nurses provide clinical and consultative services in accordance with their state nurse practice acts and the standards of the specialty. Individual roles also vary with education, experience and institutional policies.

Registered Nurse

Across the United States in diverse practice settings, RNs provide the majority of pre-travel care to travelers. Functioning within their state nurse practice acts and the standards of the specialty, they complete the pre-travel assessment of the traveler and the itinerary, identify health and safety risks of the journey, and establish with the traveler an individualized prevention plan that consists of immunizations, customized health education, and referrals as may be indicated. In many states utilizing standing orders, RNs will then proceed to vaccinate, counsel, and educate travelers about the myriad of non-vaccine-preventable risks of travel as well as travel medications ordered by prescribers in the clinical practice. RNs are also usually the first clinicians returning travelers will encounter. The RN will take a health history and triage the ill or injured traveler in accordance with practice protocols. RNs in travel health are especially alert to illness syndromes that may warrant quarantine and immediate referral for emergency care. In addition to these clinical responsibilities, RNs may function as practice managers, trainers, and members of global security, global health, emergency response, and related committees of universities, corporations, and governments. RNs contribute to travel health nursing data collection, research studies, travel health nursing guideline development, and both lay and professional publications. Individual roles also vary with education, experience, and institutional policies.

Travel Health Nurses Prepared at the Graduate Level

RNs prepared at the graduate level may assume all RN functions, augmenting the RN role within a greater range of formal training and greater authority to practice to the full extent of their education and licensure. They hold a variety of clinical and management positions. Clinical nurse specialists may serve as clinic managers and experts for orientation and training. Travel health nurses prepared at the graduate level serve as research investigators and serve on research review committees. They author professional publications (articles, chapters, texts) and also serve as peer reviewers and on journal editorial boards. In addition, these nurses may direct quality assurance efforts and oversee the development of policies and procedures. They foster collaboration with other travel health nurses and nursing organizations in the United States and elsewhere, lead efforts to establish and promote standards in the specialty and organize initiatives to develop practice innovations. The graduate-level prepared RN may serve as the clinical coordinator for vaccine trials and author travel health guidelines and regulatory content for state and national bodies such as CDC.

Advanced Practice Registered Nurse

The APRN will function, as per state regulations, either in collaboration with a physician or independently, to provide the full range of pre- and post-travel clinical services including the prescribing of medical therapies. APRNs may also qualify to provide mandated, fitness-to-travel examinations for corporate and governmental organizations as well as examinations of immigrants and refugees. These nurses may serve as tele-health clinicians assisting travelers at home and abroad, and may also serve as onsite providers accompanying traveling groups. They often have additional skills in travel disease diagnosis, management of complex cases or complicated itineraries, and the care of travelers who are pregnant, immunosuppressed, or coping with advanced illness (e.g., stage IV cancers, kidney disease requiring dialysis). In addition to these clinical roles, the APRN may be responsible for all the professional activities described for the RN and the graduate-level prepared RN. Some may also operate fully independent travel health clinics.

As travel health nursing continues to evolve and expand, nurses are assuming more varied roles within the specialty. Many travel health nurses hold graduate degrees in disciplines other than nursing (e.g., business, law, public health, epidemiology, journalism), and they utilize their specialized knowledge in a wide variety of ways—not only as clinicians, but as faculty members, informatics consultants, and department heads. They work in executive management, policy development, and as nurse leaders in nursing and multidisciplinary professional organizations. They are leaders in regional, national, and international travel health societies and organizations. They own independent practices. They write blogs and maintain a social media presence. They work in risk management and provide care to travelers in the United States and abroad.

Specialized Travel Health Nursing Education

Nurses at every educational level who practice travel health nursing find it necessary to take specialty-specific coursework in addition to the basic courses required for their state licensure as RNs or APRNs. Travel health nursing necessitates that all travel health nurses master a body of knowledge distinct from their foundational coursework of professional nursing education; travel health nursing is not routinely taught in the current registered nurse curriculum in the United States. At present, through undergraduate and graduate-level classes, short courses, CE activities, on the job mentoring, and self-directed learning, RNs acquire the knowledge and skills to provide the complete pre-travel consultation and post-travel triage. APRNs take additional courses to provide post-travel comprehensive evaluation and disease management.

Travel health nurses must know current CDC travel health and safety guidelines that include The Advisory Committee on Immunization Practices (ACIP) pre-travel vaccine recommendations and requirements, as well as destination-specific and activity-specific risks and prevention recommendations. In their clinical and administrative roles, travel health nurses understand the role and guidelines of WHO, international differences in pre- and post-travel standards, medical statistics, global health epidemiology, tropical disease transmission and avoidance, personal injury risks, behavioral health principles, transcultural considerations, and preventive and therapeutic pharmacology. Travel health nurses are familiar with specialized map reading, global geography including specific health concerns and likely activities in selected destinations, health risk analysis, individual traveler and group prevention counseling, tropical disease triage, and complex vaccination care and schedules for multiple age groups and foreign-borne travelers.

Entry into Specialty Practice

As per the *ATHNA Model Core Curriculum Guide*, foundational knowledge and skills in the specialty include:

- Knowledge and resources for national and international standards of travel health care (e.g., CDC, WHO)

- Pre-travel and post-travel assessment of the traveler and itinerary (critical questions for these consultations)

- Research methods and statistics (basic research and statistics course to comprehend and interpret the travel health literature)

- Global epidemiology of health and safety risks to the traveler (e.g., map reading, knowledge of U.S. and world geography, global disease distribution, understanding of common tourist activities in different national and world regions)

- Vaccinology (e.g., U.S. routine and travel vaccines, international immunization differences, vaccine administration requirements and documentation, issues for special travel populations such as immunocompromised, pregnancy, immigrants, and refugees)

- Behavioral measures for the prevention of travel-related injury and illness (e.g., knowledge of key prevention techniques for vector-borne diseases, motor vehicle accidents, food- and water-borne illness, personal safety, recreational hazards, climate-related risks)

- Techniques for customized, motivating health counseling designed to maximize the health and safety of diverse travelers with varied itineraries

- If not previously acquired through basic nursing education or through employment, internet search skills, cultural competency, and excellent written and verbal communication skills

- Completion of at least 20 pre-travel consultations under close supervision; more as may be necessary

- Completion of 20 post-travel triage contacts under close supervision; more as may be necessary

Continuing Education

Travel health nurses pursue any number of post-licensure educational options to build mastery and maintain currency in the specialty. Travel health nurses consult the ATHNA *Model Core Curriculum Guide*, the CDC *Health Information for International Travel*, the CDC *Epidemiology and Prevention of Vaccine Preventable Diseases*, and the *ISTM Body of Knowledge* as just four of the primary resources for acquiring and maintaining current knowledge. Additional resources include subscriptions to travel health journals, memberships in ATHNA and other travel medicine associations, ISTM and American Society of Tropical Medicine and Hygiene (ASTMH), participation in travel health webinars, courses and journal clubs, and attendance at national and international travel health, vaccinology, and tropical disease conferences. Nurses also enroll in well-established short courses developed by experts in the specialty and listed on the ATHNA *Courses and Conferences* website. Travel health risks, regulations, and therapeutic interventions change frequently, sometimes overnight, so travel health nurses recognize the necessity of ongoing education to insure quality patient care.

U.S. Nursing Programs

Comprehensive academic programs for travel health nursing in the United States continue to lag behind international learning options. To address this gap, ATHNA plans to initiate a comprehensive effort to work with U.S. nursing schools to establish 1) undergraduate courses and concentrations in travel health nursing, 2) a post-baccalaureate certificate, and 3) a graduate degree in the specialty.

Until nursing schools expand their travel health nursing curriculums, U.S. nurses entering the specialty may seek public health and tropical health degrees or complete additional academic coursework in courses such as global health, global epidemiology, tropical disease, and health coaching to supplement standard nursing courses. Many U.S. nurses take advantage of in-house training programs, enroll in several CE-accredited short courses offered year round by U.S. travel health nursing experts, and attend relevant sessions of annual conferences of American Association of Occupational Health Nurses (AAOHN), American College Health Association (ACHA), the Wilderness Medicine Society (WMS), and American Association of Nurse Practitioners (AANP). A select few U.S. nurses who seek more knowledge and skills in this specialty post-licensure may choose to undertake international courses of study such as those offered by the Faculty of Travel Medicine, Royal College of Physicians and Surgeons of Glasgow, the London School of Tropical Medicine, McGill University and the University of British Columbia.

The graduate-level prepared RN in this specialty has completed a masters, DNP, ED, or PhD program that includes academic courses in advanced research methods, statistics, epidemiology, advanced pharmacology, advanced counseling theories, and graduate-level courses in global health, tropical disease, injury prevention, and health education. Additional coursework can include any number of graduate-level management, education or clinical courses, such as health administration, finance, grant writing, project management, adult learning, advanced courses in infectious disease, courses in chronic disease management, and behavioral studies.

APRNs who practice travel health will need to complete a course of study that meets the requirements for state licensure and their professional certification (pediatrics, geriatrics, family, etc.). In addition, APRNs will need to master all the travel health knowledge and skills of the RN and take additional graduate-level courses appropriate to their role as prescribing clinician, practice director, educator, and/or researcher. APRNs who provide post-travel care will need to take advanced course work in tropical disease diagnosis and management. Language courses that facilitate communication with different travel populations are also valuable.

The *ATHNA Model Core Curriculum Guide*

Although most nursing schools offer some relevant courses, presently there are no academic centers in the United States that offer a defined nursing concentration or degree in travel health. Initially, to address this gap, ATHNA developed a travel health nursing *Model Core Curriculum Guide* that outlines the knowledge and skills required for competent practice. First written in 2002, over the years, this curriculum has served as a foundation for a number of short courses, orientation and training programs, and CE activities offered by nurse experts, travel health companies, government agencies, and academics. Posted on the ATHNA website, it is available for use by individuals and groups seeking to educate nurses in the specialty, to inform and engage many more U.S. nurses in the care of travelers, and to educate travelers about quality travel health nursing care and the specialty. This curriculum guide is periodically validated by U.S. travel health nursing experts and against other national and international curricula (e.g., ISTM Body of Knowledge, Faculty of Travel Medicine, Royal College of Physicians and Surgeons of Glasgow course) and updated regularly.

U.S. Certification in Travel Health Nursing

As of yet, no U.S. nursing certification for travel health nursing comparable to those offered by the American Nurses Credentialing Center exists. Due to this gap, some nurses have turned to alternative methods to acquire a specialty credential signifying professional development, as might be required by employment or for promotion. These nurses have applied for one of three international, interdisciplinary alternatives: the ISTM Certificate of Knowledge (CTH®), the ASTMH Certificate of Knowledge in Clinical Tropical Medicine and Travelers' Health (CTropMed®), or the Faculty of Travel Medicine, Royal College of Physicians and Surgeons of Glasgow Certification in Travel Health.

ANA recognition of the specialty of travel health nursing was the crucial first step necessary for ATHNA to pursue a certification process in alignment with other U.S. specialty nursing certifications. Not international or interdisciplinary in focus, this travel health nursing certification will be based on the U.S. standards of care and U.S. nursing regulations. The travel health nurse's attainment of this credential will document the highest skills and knowledge of travel health nursing as practiced in this country.

Commitment to Lifelong Learning

Travel health is a dynamic and ever-changing specialty. Travel health nurses are devoted to the health and education of persons and groups who travel domestically and internationally, and travel health nursing professionals focus on the multiple determinants impacting travel health that include infectious disease, environmental risks and personal safety. Travel health nursing practice "encompasses the identification and continuously changing epidemiology of travel-associated disorders and diseases and their geographical distribution, the pre-travel prevention of these conditions through education, vaccination, chemoprophylaxis, and self-treatment (for certain conditions); as well as the care of the returned ill traveler or the newly arrived migrant or refugee" (Schlagenhauf, 2010). There is really no other nursing specialty where recommendations routinely change *overnight.*

Travel health nurses know that yesterday's knowledge of global health and safety risks may not serve to protect today or tomorrow's world traveler; failure to keep current with itinerary hazards and customized risk reduction measures for the various traveling populations (e.g., students, boomers, pregnant travelers, persons with HIV, immigrants, and refugees) can result in excess travel-related illness, injury, even death.

Travel Health Nursing: Five Levels of Competency

To achieve mastery of the specialty, travel health nurses, as with other nursing specialties, progress through five levels of competency as per Benner: novice, advanced beginner, competent, proficient, and expert (Benner, 1982).

- **The Novice Travel Health Nurse**

Nurses new to travel health are novices and need careful, ongoing supervision and active mentoring as they encounter travelers in the pre- and post-travel visit for the first time. As illustrated in the *ATHNA Model Core Curriculum Guide,* travel health nursing encompasses a myriad of nursing process skills that include assessing patients, analyzing patient subjective and objective data pertinent to travel, educating patients about travel-related health risks and safety concerns, providing the correct routine, recommended and required vaccines for the patient and destination at the correct dose, as well as teaching health promotion and illness avoidance. Novice nurses need to initially observe more experienced nurses during uncomplicated encounters and then will require practice, extra time, and continuous support to provide safe and appropriate uncomplicated pre-travel consultations per clinic protocols. Novice nurses are learning with every encounter, and as learners, they have yet to acquire the requisite decision-making skills or competencies of the specialty. At this time, they must establish the habit of regularly reviewing relevant new research and updated guidelines from recognized authorities. The novice must also come to appreciate the role of the travel health nurse in bringing relevant concerns to their colleagues in their setting and broader communities for both pre- and post-travel patients.

- **The Advanced Beginner Travel Health Nurse**

The advanced beginner is a nurse who has had some experience with travel patients and so will require less direct supervision for uncomplicated traveler encounters. As travel health nursing knowledge is building, this nurse may begin, under supervision, to observe and then deliver care for more complex itineraries or travelers with special needs. This advanced beginner travel health nurse will seek out additional training beyond the core curriculum to demonstrate greater ability to research destinations for health and safety risks, to select and utilize travel health resources and references with greater ability, and to use expanded travel health and global health knowledge and vocabulary. Assessment and counseling skills continue to develop, and the advanced beginner is becoming more efficient in delivering care within the required timeframe of an encounter. This nurse must identify and begin to communicate with all relevant stakeholders including local administrators, colleagues, emergency rooms, and health departments. The advanced beginner must also become fully knowledgeable with agency policies and procedures regarding assessing and triaging patients with any post-travel concerns. There must be a focus on initial assessment and personal protective equipment, isolation procedures, appropriate referrals, and contact information for infectious disease specialists, emergency department staff, and public health departments. To gain mastery of the specialty, the advance beginner travel health nurse will ideally average 20 travelers per week for at least 1 or 2 years.

- **The Competent Travel Health Nurse**

The competent travel health nurse is a registered nurse who fully meets all the minimum competencies for the specialty and is able to provide quality pre-travel care in accordance with U.S. standards of professional nursing without additional supervision. The competent nurse demonstrates confidence, organization, and efficiency in the careful planning and delivery of pre-travel care. This nurse demonstrates the ability to utilize all available resources to increase his or her knowledge of global travel health issues and regulations. He or she is committed to self-directed learning in a specialty where travel health risks, guidelines, and recommendations can change daily. This nurse has several years of solid experience working with a variety of travelers and trip itineraries, including travelers with special needs, high-risk destinations, and hazardous travel activities. He or she has fully mastered the core curriculum for the specialty. The travel health nurse regularly collaborates and consults with primary care providers and specialists, and local public health authorities regarding any pre- and post-travel concerns. This nurse regularly engages in continuing education activities in the specialty and may have initiated or completed U.S. graduate studies relevant to travel health nursing. A competent travel health nurse may have also chosen to earn one of the international, interdisciplinary certificates from ISTM, ASTMH, the Faculty of Travel Medicine, Royal College of Physicians and Surgeons of Glasgow, or the London School of Tropical Medicine and Hygiene. He or she may be involved in local groups and committees related to travel health as well. In post-travel encounters, the competent travel health nurse, in accordance with the parameters of his or her state nursing scope of practice and institutional policies, provides triage, health evaluation, medical and nursing diagnosis, and management of health problems encountered during a domestic or international journey. The competent travel health nurse refers as appropriate and institutes a plan for follow-up care for all ill or injured travelers, including immigrants and refugees.

- **The Proficient Travel Health Nurse**

The proficient travel health nurse has gained perspective in the specialty and can anticipate with confidence the need to modify routine approaches to pre-travel care for a wide variety of travelers. Decision-making skills are highly developed, and the nurse can adjust his or her planning and care delivery to meet any time constraints. This nurse usually has 5, 10, or more years of robust experience in the specialty, has helped author practice protocols, has served to orient or mentor less experienced travel health nurses, may have participated in travel health nursing research, and may have also earned one of the international, interdisciplinary travel health certificates and/or a relevant U.S. graduate degree (e.g., MPH, MS tropical disease). Proficient travel health nurses may be involved as members or leaders in national travel health groups, organizations, and initiatives. If this nurse is also certified as an advance practice registered nurse, he or she may be examining, diagnosing, treating, and managing post-travel patients within his or her state scope of practice regulations and site guidelines. As an APRN this nurse may also provide fitness-to-travel examinations and the required evaluations of immigrants and refugees. These APRNs often serve as local experts in providing education and training of primary care staff and developing order sets and screening protocols for symptomatic as well as asymptomatic post-travelers based on current evidence-based guidelines.

- **The Expert Travel Health Nurse**

The expert travel health nurse has a deep understanding of the specialty, an intuitive grasp of travel health nursing issues, and is extremely flexible and proficient. This nurse demonstrates the highest level of analytical thinking in the specialty and is looked to by peers as a clinical authority. The expert nurse demonstrates the strongest commitment to the specialty and so will have earned a relevant graduate degree as well as one of the international, interdisciplinary certificates, and contributed to the travel health nursing research and literature. While continuing to keep current, the expert travel health nurse works to share the full breadth of his or her knowledge at the state, national, and international levels, frequently providing consulting and mentoring services, and publishing travel health-related materials outside the local practice setting. This nurse will likely be a recognized and respected leader in the specialty participating in the development of travel health nursing educational initiatives and leadership of national and international travel health organizations, both nursing and interdisciplinary.

Scope of Travel Health Nursing: The Decision Process or The HOW

Travel health nursing starts from a very broad knowledge base that includes current information regarding global epidemiology, emerging infectious diseases, human safety risks, and environmental impacts on health. This list is quite long and includes diseases from vectors, from other people, spread through contaminated food and water, associated with contact with fresh and salt water, pollution exposure, and from animal bites or stings. Travel health nurses must also be aware of threats to security, such as civil unrest and migration of refugees. One aspect that makes this role unique is the ever evolving—sometimes daily—updates that are necessary to make informed decisions. For this type of data, the travel health nurse relies on trustworthy sources such as WHO, CDC, and the Pan American Health Organization (PAHO) and specialized, commercial subscription database services. The nurse relies on updates from the U.S. State Department, the Immunization Action Coalition (IAC), and organizations such as the International Society of Travel Medicine (ISTM), the American Society of Tropical Medicine and Hygiene (ASTMH), the American Association of Occupational Health Nurses (AAOHN), the American College Health Association (ACHA), and his or her own professional association, the American Travel Health Nurses Association (ATHNA). Travel health nurses utilize content in peer-reviewed journals including the *Journal of Travel Medicine, Travel Medicine and Infectious Disease*, and the *New England Journal of Medicine*. It is also important for travel health nurses to have broad contextual knowledge around global health and traveler issues obtained from quality news sources, such as *The New York Times, National Public Radio*, and *The Wall Street Journal*.

Travel health nurses must be familiar with concerns associated with specific travel destinations and a wide variety of trip activities. They know about such hazards as air pollution, jet lag, disinsection risks (pesticide spraying of airline cabins), DVT/embolism associated with long flights or drives, barotrauma with diving, spelunking hazards, altitude sickness, frostbite, hypothermia, heat stroke/sunburn, global traffic statistics, and hazardous road conditions.

Travel health nurses must have a strong working knowledge of current immunology and vaccinology. They must understand basic principles, how to manage the cold chain and store vaccines properly, and all aspects of vaccine administration with a focus on contraindications and adverse reactions. The travel health nurse must be familiar with all U.S. routine, recommended, and required vaccines, as well as all the travel vaccines (including those available outside the United States) such as Bacille Calmette–Guerin (BCG), Japanese encephalitis, cholera, tick-borne encephalitis, rabies, typhoid, yellow fever, dengue, and Ebola. The travel health nurse keeps current with ACIP and CDC updates published in the *Weekly Morbidity and Mortality Report* (MMWR), as well as WHO and the guidelines of destination countries. Travel health nurses must also be knowledgeable about how travelers can access vaccines when traveling as well as how to complete vaccination series at reputable clinics nationally and internationally.

Often, when someone (including some health professionals) refers to travel health preparation, they describe it simply as "just getting your shots." The travel health nurse is well aware, however, that a professional, evidenced-based travel health preparation encounter is not focused on injections, but on a complex, comprehensive risk analysis that identifies clearly the specific destination risks to a particular traveler and the options available to mitigate those risks via an open dialog with the traveler in which the traveler is a full and active participant. The encounter is a complex, nuanced process that often includes immunizations, as well as extensive health counseling.

Armed with their expert knowledge base, travel health nurses complete a comprehensive assessment of each traveler and each trip. Based on the cumulative information, the travel health nurse then considers the likelihood of specific events and potential outcomes. This assessment will vary from individual to individual and trip to trip. For example, if a traveler will be staying in an urban hotel with air conditioning, the likelihood of malaria will be much lower than if the traveler is camping in a rural, high-transmission area. Another example would be exposure to Zika virus; the consequences of Zika infection for a non-pregnant traveler are usually minimal as most infections result in no symptoms. However, for a pregnant traveler the outcome of the Zika virus on the fetus can be potentially catastrophic, and is as yet, largely unknown.

For a pre-travel consultation, the travel health nurse provides any routine, recommended, and required vaccinations, medications (e.g., for traveler's diarrhea, altitude illness, leptospirosis prophylaxis, asthma, contraception), prevention and risk reduction counseling (e.g., personal safety measures, food and water precautions, insect precautions, rabies), any appropriate referrals (e.g., mental health consultation, chronic and serious illness specialists, dental care, traveler insurance), and recommendations for follow-up (e.g., fever post-travel, GI illness, booster vaccinations).

In post-travel encounters, travel health nurses will, in accordance with the parameters of their state nursing scope of practice and institutional policies, provide triage, health evaluation, medical and nursing diagnosis, and management of health problems encountered during a domestic or international journey. These problems may include trauma, routine illness, infections, and tropical or more exotic emerging diseases such as Ebola and SARS-CoV-2. The travel health nurse providing post-travel care focuses on the infectious versus the non-infectious, and proceeds to evaluate and manage the serious, treatable, and transmissible based on her level of training and practice and in accordance with site protocols, referring as appropriate. The goal is to treat the patient, while preventing transmission to others and reporting to authorities as indicated.

Scope of Travel Health Nursing: The WHY

In the United States, as well as worldwide, travel health nursing has evolved as a distinct and increasingly complex specialty over the last four decades. Travel health is devoted to the health and safety and education of persons and groups who travel nationally and internationally. Travel health nursing professionals focus on the multiple determinants impacting travel health that include infectious disease, environmental risks, and personal safety. Travel health nursing practice "encompasses the identification and continuously changing epidemiology of travel-associated disorders and diseases and their geographical distribution, the pre-travel prevention of these conditions through education, vaccination, chemoprophylaxis, and self-treatment (for certain conditions) … as well as … the care of the returned ill traveler or the newly arrived migrant or refugee" (Schlagenhauf, 2010).

The need and significance for the establishment of the travel health nursing specialty can be attributed to multiple factors: more travelers and more diversity of travelers, more travel-related illness and injury, improved epidemiology of travel-related risks, new vaccines, recognition of the critical importance of prevention counseling, recognition of the larger national and global role of travel health services, participation in the care of immigrants and refugees, and emergence of planetary health as a critical priority:

- *More travelers and more diversity of travelers*

In this century, and even more recently in the past decade, a steady, upward trend exists in the growing number and diversity of U.S. persons traveling domestically and internationally. In addition, U.S. travelers are engaged in trips with increasing duration and complexity of itineraries and travel activities. Moreover, travelers, often with complicated medical conditions and specialized equipment needed to manage those conditions, are taking journeys at all stages of life.

According to the United Nations World Tourism Organization (UNWTO) international travel increased in 2017 by 7% for a total of 1,322 billion overnight visits, a number higher than the consistent 4% annual increase since 2010. The U.S. Travel Association (USTravel.org) ranks the United States as number one for international trips taken with 21.5% of the world's total. Both groups predict that international travel will continue to increase annually by at least 4–6% in the future. More travel health nurses are needed to meet this growing demand as the destinations of travelers are also changing with increased frequency of travel to Asia, the Middle East, and Africa, placing more travelers at risk for tropical or vaccine preventable infections (CDC "Yellow Book," 2020).

- *More travel-related illness and injury*

The worldwide increase in global travel has led to more frequent exposure to illness during travel and to instances of diseases imported into the United States (e.g., measles, Zika, multidrug-resistant bacteria). Travel health nurses are prepared to provide accurate pre-travel guidance to reduce excess morbidity and mortality with age and destination appropriate vaccines and travel education. Travelers and the communities to which they return can benefit from this specialized knowledge and expertise. In addition, qualified travel health nurses provide post-travel evaluation and management services of health problems encountered during a journey. The travel health nurse providing post-travel care focuses on the infectious versus the non-infectious, and proceeds to evaluate and manage the serious, treatable, and transmissible based on his or her level of training and practice in accordance with site protocols, referring as appropriate. The goal is to treat the patient, while preventing transmission to others and reporting to institutional and public health authorities as appropriate.

- *Improved epidemiology of travel-related risks*

Over recent decades, epidemiologic studies have defined the risk for acquisition of many travel-related illnesses. Familiarity with the traveler and his or her travel details plus disease etiology and risk, prophylaxis, and self-treatment guidance have positioned the travel health nurse as the "go to" source for optimal global health related information and education. Travel health nurses now have the opportunity to aid travelers in the prevention of numerous vaccine- and non-vaccine-preventable health and safety hazards such as malaria, traveler's diarrhea, and altitude illness using medications carefully selected for efficacy, cost, and traveler preference.

- *New vaccines*

In the past 30 years, there has been tremendous growth in the field of vaccinology, with the introduction of new travel vaccines to prevent disease. Travel health nursing professionals are the most knowledgeable about the judicious use of travel vaccines such as yellow fever, typhoid, Japanese encephalitis, and cholera across the lifespan and within special populations (e.g., HIV+, pregnant, highly allergic). Travel health nurses attend expert-led educational events focused on the ever-changing ACIP immunization standards and are also well-informed about safe vaccine availability at international destinations. Travel health nurses can interpret and provide guidance with international and state vaccination records. They can assist travelers to select less risky itineraries when required vaccines are in short supply or unavailable (e.g., hepatitis A, yellow fever vaccine) or provide the traveler with international clinics where the required or recommended vaccines may be obtained safely during the journey. This often involves changing the trip timing as some immunizations require documented administration 10 days before arrival, as in the case with yellow fever.

- *Recognition of the critical importance of prevention counseling*

Health counseling to prevent illness and injury is an essential component of pre-travel care. The provision of vaccinations and chemo-prophylactic agents alone no longer meets the CDC or WHO standard for travel health prevention services. Travel health nurses discuss the impact of personal choices on travel-related illness and safety. They provide counseling on such topics as food and beverage safety, motor vehicle accident prevention, risk reduction for climate and other environmental hazards, and access to medical care here and abroad. Travel health nurses also recognize that certain travel populations have special needs and they customize their counseling for such groups, including: seniors, pregnant women, families with young children, persons with comorbidities (e.g., diabetes, CVD, migraines), persons who are highly allergic or immunosuppressed, business travelers, transgender individuals, immigrants, and refugees, and the VFR traveler who will be visiting friends and relatives.

- *Recognition of the larger national and global role of travel health nursing services*

There is recognition now that the prevention of injury and illness in travelers is only part of the much larger role of the travel health nurse. Travel health nurses serve a critical public health function as travelers and their destinations are increasingly interdependent, and are important epidemiologically because of the travelers' mobility and propensity to carry disease between countries and home. Travelers on vacation, a business trip or service project can impact the "cultural, ecological, physical, and sexual health of the local population at the travel destination" (Hill, 2006). Travel health nurses have the expertise for early identification of potential public health emergencies related to travel, and can rapidly activate public health protocols. As respected professionals in the field of travel health, travel health nurses have an important role in promoting national and global wellness by advising all travelers of evidence-based health and safety information for their current and future travel plans.

- *Participation in Immigrant and Refugee Health Services*

In 2016, more than 1 million immigrants obtained legal permanent resident status in the United States, and more than 6 million people entered the country as nonimmigrant, long-term visitors. Travel health nurses assist in health monitoring and public health communication efforts in conjunction with CDC, state, and local health departments as pertains to arriving refugees and immigrants who have notifiable health conditions. Many travel health nurses also function as contact points within the U.S. medical system for immigrants and refugees providing evaluation and ongoing care of these populations (CDC Yellow Book, 2020). Immigrants also frequently return to their country of origin to visit friends and relatives (referred to in the literature as a VFR traveler) and often erroneously assume they have natural immunity. The travel health nurse educates the immigrant traveler on his or her health risks depending on the itinerary, and will advise a post-travel appointment if additional screenings are needed to protect the traveler or the community to which he or she returns.

- *Emergence of planetary health as a critical priority*

Planetary health is a multidisciplinary field that recognizes that human health and the health of our planet are inextricably linked. Water scarcity, climate change, urbanization, changing food systems, global pollution, civil strife, and displacement have enormous implications for all of us. Travel health nurses are uniquely qualified to provide guidance to diverse travelers grappling with these concerns.

Conceptual Framework of Travel Health Nursing

The conceptual framework for travel health nursing is based on the interpersonal process in which the professional nurse launches the connection of the person to the events and situations in the environment to which they are traveling, tailors risk information based on the patient's characteristics and behaviors, and assists the patient to meet self-care needs while abroad.

The goal of the travel health nursing professional is to empower the patient to develop an accurate perception of the risk; and make clear the how, where, and when to take action, the consequences of acting or not acting; and the potential positive results of the actions selected.

Self-care is the practice of actions that individuals initiate and execute on their own behalf to maintain health and well-being. The patient's ability to engage in self-care is influenced by age, developmental state, life and travel experiences, sociocultural orientation, health status, physical abilities, and available resources. The travel health nurse assesses the patient's needs for self-care and his or her capabilities to meet those needs, while providing training and education regarding the routine, required and recommended immunizations, as well as national and global safety and security measures.

Patient

Travel health nursing is focused on assisting patients who seek travel health services. Some travelers are propelled forward into a travel health encounter by employers, school authorities, travel agents, or the military. Patients travel individually, as well as engage in groups who travel en masse or organizations that have employees or students traveling for business or educational experiences. In ways unlike other aspects of nursing, the care of the traveler also impacts the family, the community, and the world and depends on the length and destination of the journey, potential hazards encountered during travel, and the communicability of a travel-related exposure.

The travel health nursing professional performs a needs assessment, and then conveys the consequences and management of health issues and associated risks clearly so that the patient may understand the perceived severity. Travel health nursing is methodical and structured to aid domestic and international travelers to perceive severity and benefits, while exploring barriers and options. Travel health nurses explain the steps needed to take the recommended actions, while highlighting the benefits of the validated plans. Obstacles are identified and barriers to action are reduced or eliminated.

Patients are offered reassurance and assistance, even if seeking a travel health consult at the last minute, and are provided the most current information from national and international sources and experts. Travelers are often asked to participate in teach-back scenarios to demonstrate self-care skills to the travel health nurse to enhance knowledge and integrate self-efficacy.

Environment

Environment in travel health nursing has a worldwide scope. The orderly and systematic approach to this issue defines the interaction between the patient and the environment. The travel health nurse professional has to be knowledgeable about the specific patient, destinations planned, order of the trip and length of stay, social, economic, legal, and political factors involved, as well as climate, natural disasters, disease outbreaks, and the physical demands of the trip, coupled with the traveler's physical and psychological abilities. Additionally, the patient must be informed about emergency medical care, trip insurance for medical evacuation, if needed, and local clinics where linguistics would not be a barrier. Advances in scientific knowledge and tele-health technology also impact the traveling public domain with up-to-the-minute access to advice, interventions, and responses. Finally, general conditions such as cultural considerations, food and fluids safety, transportation methods, and air/water pollution must be taken into account, so travelers know when and how to seek appropriate medical assistance.

Travel Health Nursing Professional

Travel health nursing professionals are a cluster of specially educated and trained registered nurses, graduate-level prepared nurses and advanced practice registered nurses who exercise expert nursing process skills of assessing patients, analyzing patient subjective and objective data pertinent to travel, educating about domestic and international health risks and safety concerns, and teaching health promotion and illness avoidance. The methods are evidence-based and in accordance with professional and ethical standards. Travel health nurses practice within the scope of their state nurse practice acts and the standards of the specialty. They function as direct care providers, consultants to businesses and the traveling public, researchers, faculty members, and nursing leaders. Many are entrepreneurs, serving as owners and operators of their own travel health centers. The travel health nursing professional is a strong patient advocate for those traveling domestically and abroad, ensuring that the trip planned is physically possible for the traveler (e.g. an elderly couple who wish to trek through the Amazon may be better served on a cruise ship where medical services have a presence). Essential to the encounter is the use of age-appropriate and evidence-based nursing assessments, followed by detailed documentation of the visit, including immunizations and trip guidance.

ATHNA's Travel Health Nursing Conceptual Framework

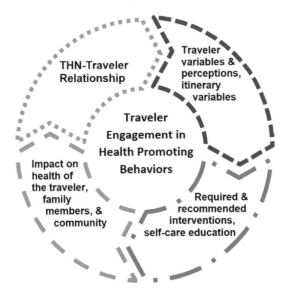

Application of Code of Ethics Provisions by Travel Health Nurses

ANA's *Code of Ethics for Nurses with Interpretive Statements* is applicable for all nurses. The following discussion of the nine provisions clarifies its relevance to travel health nursing.

Provision 1: The nurse practices with compassion and respect for the inherent dignity, worth, and unique attributes of every person. (ANA, 2015)

The travel health nurse strives to assist the traveler to achieve maximum health and safety during and after international and domestic journeys. Travel health nurses provide care to travelers regardless of socio-economic status, immigration status, health status, culture, values, religious or spiritual beliefs, sexual orientation, language, race, gender, or age. Every individual is treated with respect during the pre- and post-travel encounter. When assessing itinerary risks, travel health nurses have an ethical responsibility to have a clear understanding of travel-related health and safety risks of specific populations including, but not limited to, patients who are pregnant, pediatric travelers, seniors, immunosuppressed patients, patients with severe allergies, and immigrants and refugees who return home to visit friends and relatives (i.e. VFR traveler). Travel health nurses set aside biases and prejudices with regard to the purpose of travel, timing of the pre-travel visit, destination choice, or planned trip activities. The basic ethical tenets of autonomy and informed consent are essential in providing individualized education and resources to mitigate travel-related risks that are often numerous and may include food and water pathogens, insect vector diseases, air quality threats, societal unrest and infectious outbreaks. The travel health nurse always supports the self-care agency of travelers and their right to self-determination as it applies to risk reduction interventions (e.g., immunizations, medications, referrals, change of itinerary). In the post-travel encounter, the travel health nurse withholds judgment regarding the circumstances of the post-travel illness or injury, and acts in the interest of the patient and other stakeholders in a caring and compassionate manner.

Provision 2: The nurse's primary commitment is to the patient, whether an individual, family, group, community, or population.

Travel health nurses are central to preparing travelers in a variety of circumstances: solo business travelers, immigrant families returning home to visit friends and relatives, researchers, mission and humanitarian workers, students traveling abroad, patients seeking international medical care, and military personnel, among others. Increasingly, travel health nurses also evaluate and manage the care of the ill or injured returning traveler consistent with their scope of practice and applicable regulations. To assure the highest quality care, travel health nurses reject conflicts of interest and use evidence-based recommendations and interventions free of commercial bias. Travel health nurses prioritize not only individual patients but also the broader population, utilizing a public health perspective to protect the communities both at home and abroad. Travel health nurses work to prevent future epidemics (e.g. advising patients to use insect precautions to circumvent infecting local vectors) and minimize the spread of infectious diseases (e.g., instructing travelers to seek care immediately when they develop fever if at risk of malaria, viral hemorrhagic fever, MERS, avian influenza etc., discouraging unvaccinated travelers from infecting local populations abroad with measles or other illnesses, and rapidly reporting communicable diseases to the appropriate authorities).

Provision 3: The nurse promotes, advocates for, and protects the rights, health, and safety of the patient.

During the pre-travel encounter, the role of the travel health nurse is to implement travel health consultations and raise awareness of health and safety risks related to domestic and international travel. Utilizing customized assessment tools and a variety of reliable resources (e.g., CDC, WHO, the Pan American Health Organization), travel health nurses conduct a thorough risk assessment of all aspects of the individual traveler and the trip, including the complete itinerary and planned activities. Travel health nurses then develop a customized plan encompassing evidenced-based personal safety measures, food and water precautions, insect precautions, appropriate vaccines, medications, and a follow-up care plan to mitigate risks. The travel health nurse administers vaccines in a correct and safe manner, in accordance with CDC, state and institutional guidelines, having fully informed the patient and obtained consent. During a post-travel encounter, the travel health nurse ensures that returning travelers receive any appropriate follow-up care, including completing a vaccine series, triage or evaluation and management in the event of any rabies exposure, post-travel illness, or injury. In addition, responsibility for the patient does not end with referral to a specialist team. The travel health nurse ensures that the transition of care is complete, and follows the patient to the extent feasible or possible throughout the healing process.

Provision 4: The nurse has authority, accountability, and responsibility for nursing practice, makes decisions, and takes action consistent with the obligation to promote health and to provide optimal care.

Travel health nursing professionals take responsibility for all aspects of their practice. Travel health nurses are knowledgeable regarding respective nurse practice acts, federal guidelines, and organizational policies, and the *ANA Code of Ethics for Nurses with Interpretive Statements*. They identify any unmet needs and ensure appropriate follow-up. They coordinate with other health care team members and bring attention to any inconsistencies or outdated practices. In their care of the traveler and their interactions with colleagues, they adhere to the *Travel Health Nursing: Scope and Standards of Practice, 1st edition (2021)*. They keep current with frequent changes in global health patterns that impact their care, seeking information from only reliable sources, completing CE courses, complying with state, local, and national regulatory bodies including those for nursing and public health. They regularly evaluate their care, and update their recommendations based on guidance from agencies, such as the WHO and CDC.

Provision 5: The nurse owes the same duties to self as to others, including the responsibility to promote health and safety, preserve wholeness of character and integrity, maintain competence, and continue personal and professional growth.

Travel health nurses may function in settings with unique risks to their health and safety. They may work abroad in limited resource settings or practice in clinics involving exposure to post-travel patients with infectious diseases, such as avian influenza, MERS, or viral hemorrhagic fevers, such as Ebola. Moral distress occurs when travel health nurses encounter barriers to care or travelers who received pre-travel care inconsistent with U.S. standards. Travel health nurses must have the moral self-respect and courage to deal with these situations with patient education and advocacy and, as may be indicated, mandatory reporting or professional referrals in-country or abroad. Travel health nurses often collaborate in settings (e.g., universities, corporations, public health departments) that pose ethical dilemmas concerning the availability and extent of pre-travel services and the adequate financing of those services. Knowledge of state nurse practice acts, CDC travel health guidelines, current travel health research, and global illness and injury epidemiology enables the travel health nurse to demonstrate the expertise and leadership required to ensure comprehensive, quality care for every traveler. Expectations of others may exceed the travel health nurse's scope of practice and thereby jeopardize the health and welfare of travelers, colleagues, and travel health nurses themselves. The travel health nurse maintains self-respect in terms of expectations for adequate orientation and training, time for counseling, access to necessary resources, and use of colleagues for collaboration. Travel health nurses have an ethical responsibility to follow evidence-based recommendations to maintain their health and safety both at work and outside the workplace.

Travel health nurses also must not fall prey to conflicts of interest that compromise character and integrity. They must not engage in personal or professional relationships that adversely influence the quality of care they provide. For example, they may not profit from recommending unnecessary vaccines or skewing research results. Travel health nurses carry the special burden of working in a rapidly changing field—daily updates are usually needed to track epidemiological changes in current outbreaks and emerging infectious diseases. Travel health nurses must seek information only from reliable sources, such as the CDC and WHO. They must avail themselves regularly of CE programs that focus on a variety of areas including tropical medicine, global health, climate change, epidemiology, immunology/vaccinology, and pre-travel consultation and communication. Finally, travel health nurses ensure continued growth and development through participation in professional organizations such as the American Travel Health Nurses Association, the International Society of Travel Medicine and the American Society of Tropical Medicine and Hygiene.

Provision 6: The nurse, through individual and collective effort, establishes, maintains, and improves the ethical environment of the work setting and conditions of employment that are conducive to safe, quality health care.

Travel health nurses, working in concert with other health professionals and relevant stakeholders, operate in a myriad of roles to promote ethics in the workplace and ensure high-quality care. Travel health nursing professionals are clinicians, academic researchers, educators, public health officials, executives, and national, as well as international, policy developers. They participate in quality assurance activities, such as chart review, evaluation of services using outcome measures, and patient surveys. They implement policies that prevent commercial interests, such as pharmaceutical companies, from adversely influencing their work. They develop and seek out evidenced-based interventions (e.g., ACIP vaccine recommendations). They work across disciplines and utilize the latest technological developments to eliminate obstacles, improve access to care, eliminate inefficiencies, reduce costs, and enhance quality of care.

Provision 7: The nurse, in all roles and settings, advances the profession through research and scholarly inquiry, professional standards development, and generation of both nursing and health policy.

Travel health nurses advance the specialty by integrating evidence-based findings into practice, taking on projects, serving on committees, and assuming leadership positions within their own organizations, as well as outside institutions. They initiate, promote, and collaborate on research endeavors through academic institutions, professional societies and organizations, such as the American Travel Health Nurses Association, International Society of Travel Medicine, American College Health Association, American Association of Occupational Health Nurses, the U.S. Armed Forces, and Centers for Disease Control and Prevention. They work across disciplines, including tropical medicine, infectious disease, public health, pharmacy, and veterinary medicine, to ensure that travel health nurses have a seat at the table to shape policies affecting their patients. They advocate at their workplace and in the public arena for improved care to international travelers utilizing the *Travel Health Nursing: Scope and Standards of Practice, 1st edition (2021)*.

Provision 8: The nurse collaborates with other health professionals and the public to protect human rights, promote health diplomacy, and reduce health disparities.

Travel health nurses have an ethical responsibility to engage in activities that promote and protect the dignity and basic rights of all individuals. Health is a universal right and travel health nurses work every day to make it a high national and international priority. Travel health nurses collaborate across a wide variety of disciplines to promote health individually, locally, and globally through institutional projects and committees, community action and consumer groups, as well as legislative and policy work. They give presentations, conduct research, teach and mentor colleagues, engage in legislative efforts and effectively utilize print, broadcast, and social media to address concerns. They address such disparities as access to pre- and post-travel care, providing accurate and evidenced-based information on immunizations, preventing and controlling infectious diseases and their responsible vectors, and addressing the impact of climate change on global health and infectious disease. They also address world-wide accident prevention, especially the high rates of motor vehicle accidents, ensuring reproductive rights by providing safe and effective methods of contraception, and mitigating, to the extent possible, sexual assault, human trafficking, exploitation, and travel concerns of vulnerable populations including, but not limited to, the LGBTQ+ community, immigrants and refugees, and travelers with physical disabilities or mental illness.

Provision 9: The profession of nursing, collectively through its professional organizations, must articulate nursing values, maintain the integrity of the profession, and integrate principles of social justice into nursing and health policy.

Nurses have a long tradition of being formidable advocates for change, and nurses working collectively can be even more effective change agents. There is power in numbers, and travel health nurses working with their professional organizations to articulate nursing values and health priorities can improve the health and well-being of patients and communities worldwide.

The values of travel health nursing professionals are advanced broadly and communicated widely through the American Travel Health Nurses Association (ATHNA) and its membership. This professional association serves as a conduit to maintain and further the integrity of the specialty practice. It works to align the guiding principles of evidence-based practice with those of social justice and integrate them into nursing policy. ATHNA provides travel health nurses with ready access to the latest clinical updates, courses and conferences, specialized standing orders, and other online resources that support this effort. The association promotes personal and global health and safety, as well as research integrity, and regularly identifies and addresses weaknesses in travel health care delivery. ATHNA highlights the special concerns of specific populations of travelers to enhance the quality of care for all.

Travel health nurses serve as experts to guide decisions involving travel health care both in the United States and internationally. They establish education requirements, standards of care, health policy and national and international health agendas. Travel health nurses, acting through ATHNA, are strong advocates for the profession as illustrated by their recent success in convincing CDC to avoid using "travel health physician" in their publications, replacing this with more inclusive terms such as travel health "professional" or "clinician" to more accurately reflect the role of nurses as travel health experts. Travel health nurses, acting through ATHNA, are strong advocates for the profession as also illustrated by the successful ATHNA effort to achieve ANA recognition of travel heath nursing as a specialty practice of professional nursing.

Historical Perspective: The Specialty of Travel Health Nursing

While there have always been travelers and clinicians willing to help prepare them for their journeys, travel medicine evolved as a U.S. medical specialty in the 1980s. Initially, the specialty was known as "Emporiatrics," and the number of providers grew as U.S. businesses expanded globally, tourism increased, and more students elected to study abroad.

Travel health nursing developed in parallel to travel medicine. During the 1980s, nurses in college health, occupational health, and ambulatory care were called upon to add pre-travel assessment and risk management services to their clinical role. At first, these nurses supported physicians in the care of patients traveling internationally, but by the late 1980s, nurses started to assume central roles in the preparation of all travelers. These nurses came from many different professional nursing backgrounds, but soon they all self-identified as travel health nurses. Often confused by the public as nurses who traveled from hospital to hospital for seasonal or temporary employment ("traveling nurses"), travel health nursing professionals brought a strong commitment to prevention and quality care to their practice of preparing business and personal travelers. Of necessity, they were all self-taught since no travel medicine textbooks existed, the CDC "Yellow Book" was only a small pamphlet, and nursing schools offered little curricula specific to travel health.

In 1991, physicians and nurses from around the world met in Atlanta to form an international, interdisciplinary professional organization, the International Society of Travel Medicine (ISTM). More than 600 nurses in attendance voted for a more inclusive name; however, when these nurses left the meeting, there was already consensus that U.S. nurses needed to form their own network for support, education, and professional development. Informal groups started to spring up around the country and then, in 1999, the New York Nurses Network was established. This self-funded group, initially comprised of 25 nurses, met six to eight times a year for case studies, clinical updates, and professional networking. At the same time, principals in the New York group also started a nursing task force within ISTM, joined ISTM committees, and presented posters at biennial international meetings. At these meetings in Paris, Lisbon, and Montreal, they learned about travel health nurses coming together as a national specialty in the United Kingdom and in the Netherlands, and soon they, too, started to envision a travel health nursing specialty in the United States.

By 2004, the New York Network had seriously outgrown its name and now included nurses from around the country; the necessity and benefit for creating a national professional travel health nursing organization was apparent. With that in mind, ATHNA was incorporated in 2004 and established as a tax-exempt entity under Section 501(c) (3) of the U.S. Internal Revenue Service Code and registered with the NYS Attorney General's Charities Bureau. As described in the articles of incorporation, "This Corporation is formed to advance the profession of travel health nurses. Its purpose is educational within the meaning of 501(c) (3) of the Internal Revenue Code, including, but not limited to, the advancement of travel health nursing through education and public awareness." ATHNA's inaugural board included founding members from the New York Network, as well as nurses from Wisconsin, California, Colorado, Texas, Massachusetts, and New Hampshire.

From its inception, ATHNA was committed to the inclusion of all nurses (RNs, graduate-level prepared nurses, APRNs) who provided care to travelers; the organization reached out to nurses working in college health, occupational health, public health, the military, private practice, and academic centers. In its earliest years, ATHNA was not yet a full-fledge membership society, but rather ATHNA saw its purpose to serve as a primary professional resource for U.S. nurses entering the field and as an engine for professional development and advocacy for the specialty of travel health nursing in this country.

With those goals in mind, ATHNA established an open-access website for communication (www.athna.org), wrote the first *Travel Health Nursing: Scope & Standards of Practice (2004)* and stated its mission as: "The Mission of ATHNA is the advancement of the profession of travel health nurses through education and public awareness." On its fifth anniversary as a professional society, ATHNA voted to expand into a membership organization. That goal was fully achieved on April 15, 2010.

Since that time, ATHNA has continued to grow its numbers and expand its support for travel health nursing. Today, more than 2,200 nurses representing every state, as well as other nations, are registered members. To promote networking and keep travel health nurses updated, ATHNA continues to add website content, including a Clinic Manual, Clinic Toolkit, standing order templates, updated listing of *Courses and Conferences*, a *CareerCenter*, as well as links to CDC and the International Association for Medical Assistance to Travelers (IAMAT). Regular educational features include a monthly Constant Contact communication, the ATHNA blog *TravelBytes* and the Q&A column *Ask Us Anything*. Since 2010, ATHNA has offered a variety of CE activities that now includes its unique and innovative annual NED: Networking, Education, and Development Day. This free member benefit is a novel CE activity offered simultaneously each summer in multiple U.S. communities. In 2018, members attended NED sessions in California, New York, Texas, and Pennsylvania. In addition, ATHNA provides periodic free or low-cost CE accredited content on its website. To support comprehensive and quality travel health nursing education consistent with U.S. standards, ATHNA has also created and posted on its website a *Model Core Curriculum Guide* for nurses entering the specialty and for the development of short courses, CE activities, and nursing school courses, concentrations, post-baccalaureate certificates, and graduate degrees in the specialty.

Since its founding, ATHNA has been a strong advocate for travel heath nursing research and its *Travel Well Research Award* has been conferred several times over the past decade. ATHNA facilitates the collaboration of members on studies that benefit travel health nursing as a specialty, as well as studies to improve traveler outcomes. Recently, ATHNA members were awarded first prize for their ISTM poster "The Highly Allergic Traveler: Simple Steps to Save a Life." Currently, ATHNA is partnering with CDC, ISTM and ACHA on a multi-site, multi-year study of student travel health.

ATHNA created a working group in 2012 to explore official recognition of travel health nursing as a specialty. In 2017, the ATHNA Board of Directors met in retreat to develop a 5-year strategic plan that included an updated mission statement and established the goal of ANA specialty recognition as a priority. A proposal to create an ATHNA Fellows program was launched, and a plan for the first national ATHNA meeting was initiated. The Board also made a commitment to foster certification in alignment with U.S. standards for travel health nurses and to encourage academic courses, concentrations and degrees in the specialty. The mission of ATHNA was updated to reflect these goals: "The mission of the American Travel Health Nurses Association is to advance nurses engaged in the care of travelers through professional development, evidence-based practice and advocacy." The inaugural class of ATHNA Fellows, ten outstanding contributors to the science and development of travel health nursing, was introduced at the well-received first national ATHNA meeting held on June 4, 2019 at the Barbara Jordan Conference Center in Washington, DC. Conference attendees expressed the universal hope that this meeting might become an annual event.

Future Trends

Travel health nursing is a dynamic and rapidly evolving specialty because of numerous and ever-changing factors that impact the traveling public such as vaccine-preventable diseases and the availability of routine, recommended, or required vaccines; non-vaccine-preventable diseases that spread without warning over a large geographical region or regions, the age, gender, health, physical and psychological capabilities of the traveler, and the purpose of the trip, including planned activities, season, political climate, and potential for extreme weather hazards. At present, travel health nurses have concerns about inconsistencies in the delivery of pre- and post-travel nursing care, questions about patient safety, concerns about the undue influence of pharmaceutical representatives and potential conflicts of interest in for-profit settings, as well as the lack of training opportunities in travel health nursing. Travel health nurses are frustrated by vaccine shortages and inadequate insurance coverage for prevention services; they are eager for more evidence-based recommendations, and they bemoan the public's lack of understanding about what constitutes a comprehensive, quality pre-travel encounter (it is so much more than "just shots"). Unfortunately, travel health nurses also face frequent challenges regarding the lack of travel health training and knowledge that still exists among primary care providers and specialists.

It is anticipated that the future of travel health nursing will include even more travel and more traveler diversity, advancing technology, planetary health components, vaccine considerations, cost containment issues, expanding role for the nursing profession, recognition of the larger global role of travel health nursing services, expansion of ATHNA, establishment of U.S. travel health nursing post-baccalaureate certificates and graduate degrees, and U.S. travel health nursing certification.

Even more travel and more diverse travelers: According to CDC (2017), Americans of all ages made more than 73 million trips internationally in 2015; that number is expected to increase by 4% to 7% annually as more citizens are traveling for business, education, pleasure, volunteerism, health care, or to visit friends and relatives. More than one billion people traveled worldwide internationally in 2017, and approximately 50% became ill or injured while overseas. Furthermore, some travelers required medical care upon arriving home (Keystone et al., 2013).

As more people travel this country and the world, the need for skilled travel health nurses and pre-travel health services will be critical in providing travelers with health and safety information specific to their particular needs and destinations. Additionally, travel health nurses will be increasingly able to offer traveling patients effective and specialized in-transit care using advanced technology and access to collegial resources in all parts of the nation and the world. There will also be an increased need for travel health nurses prepared to deliver post-travel care to the greater number of travelers expected to return home ill or injured. Much of this care requires the specialized education and training of the travel health nurse and is generally not available in primary care offices or urgent care centers.

Advancing technology: Technology across all health specialties is increasing and travel health is benefitting from this innovation. In coming years specific considerations for the travel health nurse will include how best to assist the traveler with access to more travel apps and alerts, and ready access to electronic health and immunization records, both domestic and international. The travel health nurse will have opportunities to utilize technology to decrease costs and provide higher quality services via video/tele-health visits and to access point-of-service labs and other diagnostics as needed.

Planetary health: Travel health nurses already recognize that the health of individuals is interdependent with the health of animals and the environment. According to CDC, "One Health is defined as a collaborative, multi-sectoral, and trans-disciplinary approach—working at the local, regional, national, and global levels—with the goal of achieving optimal health outcomes, recognizing the interconnection between people, animals, plants, and their shared environment (CDC, 2017)." It will be increasingly essential that travel health nurses collaborate and coordinate with professionals from veterinary medicine, environmental groups, public health, the law, etc. It is likely that ongoing climate change will bring with it new and emerging infectious diseases, as well as serious, non-infectious, and chronic illnesses, such as pollution-related exposures that could affect travelers going to any destination.

Vaccine considerations: Vaccines are considered one of the cornerstones in preventing some of the most common illnesses encountered in global travel, including predictable disease and exotic syndromes. While new vaccines continue to be developed, availability, efficacy, safety, cost, and acceptability will remain issues for both the traveling public and travel health nurses alike.

Cost containment issues: Travel health nurses will need to find innovative ways to effectively engage stakeholders and provide high-quality services in ways that are affordable and sustainable for all travelers.

Expanding role for the nursing profession: As reported by the Robert Wood Johnson Foundation in its 2019 report, "Activating Nursing to Address Unmet Need in the 21st Century," nurses will increasingly have a larger role in meeting the health needs of individuals and populations. With their global knowledge and perspective, travel health nurses will have more opportunities to contribute to the public health of this country and others. Travel health nurses' knowledge of vaccines, global diseases (e.g., Ebola, MERS, COVID-19, avian flu, and measles) and WHO international health regulations (IHR) can assist governments, corporations, universities, and others with the prevention of local outbreaks, stigma, and fear.

Recognition of the larger global role of travel health nursing services: There is growing recognition that the prevention of injury and illness in travelers is only part of the much larger role of the travel health nurse. Travel health nurses serve a critical public health function as travelers and the destinations to which they journey are increasingly interdependent, and travelers are important epidemiologically because of their mobility and propensity to carry disease between countries and home. Travelers on vacation, a business trip or service project can impact the "cultural, ecological, physical, and sexual health of the local population at the travel destination (Hill, 2006)." Travel health nurses have the expertise for early identification of potential public health emergencies related to travel, and can rapidly activate public health protocols. As respected professionals in the field of travel health, travel health nurses have an important role in promoting global wellness by advising travelers of evidence-based health and safety information for their current and future travel plans.

Expansion of ATHNA: As estimated by CDC and others, more than 25,000 nurses now provide travel health services in a variety of settings around the United States. ATHNA will continue to expand its membership and mission to represent the varied interests, work sites, educational, and professional needs of travel health nurses. ATHNA will also enhance its collaboration with other major international organizations for travel health, including ISTM, ACHA, AAOHN, and ASTMH. One ongoing initiative is the joint Student Travel Abroad research project with CDC, ACHA, ISTM, and ATHNA.

U.S. travel health nursing education: As domestic and international travel increases and more nurses participate in pre- and post-travel care, the need for travel health nursing curricula will grow. ATHNA will continue to offer relevant CE programs, revise and promote its website-based *Model Core Curriculum Guide,* and continue its efforts for the inclusion of travel health nursing content in undergraduate and graduate nursing education with more courses, as well as a travel health nursing concentration, a post-baccalaureate certificate, and graduate degrees in the specialty.

U.S. travel health nursing certification: Lacking a U.S. equivalent, a small number of travel health nurses who seek a specialty credential for professional development, employment, or promotion currently apply for one of three international, interdisciplinary alternatives: the ISTM Certificate of Knowledge (CTH®), the ASTMH Certificate of Knowledge in Clinical Tropical Medicine and Travelers' Health (CTropMed®), or the Faculty of Travel Medicine, Royal College of Physicians and Surgeons of Glasgow Certification in Travel Health. However, none of these are specific to professional nursing, nor do they confirm knowledge or compliance with U.S. standards of nursing or travel health care. In addition, none adhere to the eligibility or renewal criteria typical of any American Nurses Credentialing Center (ANCC) certifications. Travel health nurses are asking for U.S. certification, and ATHNA will continue to explore options for establishing a certification in travel health nursing consistent with other professional nursing certifications recognized in this country.

The future will pose significant challenges, but travel health nurses are in a unique position to address these concerns, ensure travelers receive the highest-quality care, and protect the communities to which travelers visit and return. Travel health nurses will meet these challenges in several key respects by:

- Aligning U. S. travel health nurses with medical, pharmacy, and international nursing organizations specializing in travel health

- Increasing the publication of evidence-based travel health and travel health nursing research

- Providing new health career options for nursing students and expanding undergraduate and graduate curricula to include travel nursing health topics and concentrations utilizing the ATHNA *Model Core Curriculum Guide*

- Ensuring nursing professionalism with a code of ethics specific to travel health nursing practice

Standards of Travel Health Nursing Practice

Standard 1. Assessment

The travel health nurse collects comprehensive data and information regarding the traveler and the trip.

Competencies

The travel health nurse:

- ▶ Collects comprehensive data including, but not limited to, physical, functional, psychosocial, emotional, cognitive, sexual, cultural, age-related, temporal, environmental, spiritual/transpersonal, and economic assessments in a systematic and ongoing process while honoring the uniqueness of the traveler.

- ▶ Elicits the traveler's values, preferences, personal attitudes, beliefs, expressed needs, and knowledge of the journey.

- ▶ Involves the traveler, other stakeholders as appropriate, in holistic data collection and shared decision-making.

- ▶ Identifies barriers (e.g., psychosocial, literacy, financial, cultural, temporal) to effective communication and comprehensive data collection.

- ▶ Makes appropriate adaptations to ensure effective communication and comprehensive data collection as may be indicated.

- ▶ Prioritizes the assessment of health and safety risks to the traveler based on geographic areas, modes of transportation, duration of travel, accommodations, and other itinerary factors. (In post-travel scenarios, the health and safety risks to other staff and the broader community must also be considered).

- Uses evidence-based principles, models, and tools of epidemiology, demography, and biostatistics, as well as social, behavioral, and natural and applied sciences to structure data collection.

- Prioritizes data collection activities based on assessment parameters identified by CDC, WHO, and experts in the field as well as the anticipated needs of the traveler or itinerary.

- Synthesizes available data, information, and knowledge relevant to the traveler and itinerary to identify patterns of travel and individual variances.

- Applies relevant governmental requirements, ethical standards, and institutional privacy guidelines to the collection, maintenance, use, and dissemination of data and information.

- Recognizes the traveler as the authority on his or her own health by respecting his or her own preferences.

- Documents data in a retrievable format.

Additional Competencies for the Graduate-Level Prepared Travel Health Nurse and APRN

The graduate-level prepared travel nurse:

- Assesses the effect of health and travel interactions among individuals, family, community, and social systems on health and illness.

- Gathers data from multiple, interdisciplinary sources using appropriate methods to augment and/or verify population-focused data.

- Synthesizes population-focused data from multiple sources throughout the assessment process.

Additional Competencies for the Advance Practice Registered Nurse (APRN)

In addition to the competencies of the registered nurse and the graduate-level prepared registered nurse, the advanced practice registered nurse:

- Initiates diagnostic tests and procedures relevant to the traveler's current health status.

- Uses advanced assessment, knowledge, and skills to maintain, enhance, or improve health conditions.

Standard 2. Diagnosis

The travel health nurse analyzes the assessment data to determine diagnoses and travel-related risks and issues.

Competencies

The travel health nurse:

- ▶ Derives the diagnoses and travel-related health and safety risks and issues through an analysis of a broad range of assessment data, including data from the traveler.

- ▶ Validates the diagnoses and travel-related risks and issues with the traveler and other healthcare providers when possible and appropriate.

- ▶ Identifies actual or potential risks to the traveler's health and safety that may include, but are not limited to, interpersonal, systematic, temporal, or environmental circumstances. (In post-travel scenarios, the health and safety risks to other staff and the broader community must also be considered).

- ▶ Uses standardized classification systems and clinical support tools, when available, in identifying diagnoses and issues.

- ▶ Documents diagnoses or travel-related risks and issues in a manner that facilitates the determination of the expected outcomes and plan.

- ▶ Bases the analysis on current research and knowledge in travel health nursing and medicine relevant to potential problem areas.

- ▶ Selects diagnoses relevant to the travel population.

- ▶ Explains the diagnoses or travel-related risks and issues to the traveler.

Additional Competencies for the Graduate-Level Prepared Travel Health Nurse

The graduate-level prepared travel health nurse:

- ▶ Supports staff in developing and maintaining competency in the diagnostic process.

- ▶ Provides education and resources to assist nurses to develop and utilize travel health diagnoses.

▶ Contributes to global disease surveillance research through diagnostic data analysis.

Additional Competencies for the APRN

In addition to the competencies of the registered nurse and the graduate-level prepared registered nurse, the advanced practice registered nurse:

▶ Systematically compares and contrasts clinical findings, such as laboratory results, with normal and abnormal variations in formulating a differential diagnosis.

▶ Utilizes complex data and information obtained during interview, examination, and diagnostic processes in identifying diagnoses.

Standard 3. Outcomes Identification

The travel health nurse identifies expected outcomes for a plan individualized to the traveler and the itinerary.

Competencies

The travel health nurse:

▶ Involves the traveler and others in formulating expected outcomes when possible and appropriate.

▶ Derives culturally appropriate expected outcomes from the diagnoses.

▶ Considers associated risks, benefits, costs, current scientific evidence, and clinical expertise when formulating expected outcomes.

▶ Defines expected outcomes in terms of the traveler, the traveler's culture and values, ethical and environmental considerations, and the itinerary.

▶ Includes a time and financial estimate for the attainment of expected outcomes.

▶ Develops expected outcomes that facilitate continuity of care.

▶ Identifies expected outcomes according to changes in the status of the traveler or evaluation of the traveler's needs or concerns, or availability of resources.

▶ Documents expected outcomes as measurable goals.

▶ Acts as a resource for the travel health community in the development of individual health and safety outcome plans.

▶ Uses standardized language or internationally recognizable terminology to document the outcome in a retrievable form.

▶ Identifies expected outcomes that incorporate scientific evidence and are achievable through implementation of evidence-based practices.

▶ Recognizes expected outcomes that address cost-effectiveness and clinical effectiveness, traveler satisfaction, and continuity and consistency among providers.

▶ Differentiates outcomes that require care process interventions from those that require system-level interventions.

Additional Competencies for the Graduate-Level Prepared Travel Health Nurse and the APRN

The graduate-level prepared travel health nurse or the advanced practice registered nurse:

▶ Acts a resource for the travel health community in the development of population-based health and safety outcomes.

▶ Identifies trends in travel health outcomes to guide clinical planning for future travel health programs.

Standard 4. Planning
The travel health nurse develops a plan that prescribes strategies and alternatives to attain expected, measurable outcomes.

Competencies

▶ Develops an individualized plan in partnership with the traveler and others considering the person's characteristics or itinerary, including but not limited to values, beliefs, spiritual and health practices, preferences, developmental level, coping style, culture, environment, dates of travel, style of travel, accommodations, transportation, and available technology.

▶ Uses diagnostic test findings to guide interventions relevant to the traveler's current status.

▶ Prioritizes the plan of care with the traveler and others as appropriate.

▶ Includes strategies that address each of the identified diagnoses including potential emergency plans. These may include, but are not limited to, strategies for:

- Promotion and restoration of health;

- Prevention of illness (chronic and acute), injury, and disease (both routine and exotic);

- The alleviation of suffering; and

- Emergency preparedness and response (outbreaks, travel medical insurance, U.S. resources and resources at destination, post-travel public health concerns, etc.).

▶ Modifies the plan incorporating as appropriate health behavior change theory, new knowledge, traveler response, or other relevant factors to enhance implementation and achieve expected outcomes.

▶ Provides for continuity in the plan (including opportunities to adjust the plan at destination if needed).

▶ Incorporates an implementation pathway or timeline in the plan.

▶ Considers the economic impact of the plan on the traveler and other affected parties.

- ▶ Integrates current and emerging trends and research in nursing and travel health-related fields in the planning process.

- ▶ Utilizes the plan to provide direction to other members of the healthcare team.

- ▶ Ensures adequate space, time, information resources, and privacy for the travel health nurse and the traveler to explore suggested, potential, and alternative options.

- ▶ Defines the plan to reflect current statutes, rules and regulations, and standards.

- ▶ Modifies the plan according to the ongoing assessment of the traveler's response, current outbreaks, and other outcome indicators.

- ▶ Documents the plan in a manner that uses standardized language and internationally recognized terminology, that is culturally sensitive, and is at an appropriate reading level.

- ▶ Identifies assessment and diagnostic strategies and therapeutic interventions that reflect current evidence, including data, research, literature, and expert nursing and travel health knowledge.

- ▶ Designs strategies to meet the multifaceted needs of travelers with complex healthcare needs.

- ▶ Includes the synthesis of traveler values and beliefs regarding nursing and medical therapies in the plan.

- ▶ Uses an ecological perspective in planning.

- ▶ Provides for continuity within and across programs and services.

Additional Competencies for the Graduate-Level Prepared Travel Health Nurse and the APRN

The graduate-level prepared travel health nurse or the advanced practice registered nurse:

▶ Leads the design and development of processes that include the use of other health professionals to address the identified diagnoses.

▶ Actively participates in the development and continuous improvement of systems that support the planning process.

▶ Participates in the integration of fiscal, human, material, population, and scientific resources to enhance and complete the planning process for travel health programs or services.

Standard 5. Implementation

The travel health nurse implements the identified plan.

Competencies

The travel health nurse:

- ▶ Partners with the traveler and others as appropriate to implement the plan in a safe, realistic, timely, and cost-effective manner.

- ▶ Provides care to diverse travel populations over the lifespan that is empathetic, culturally competent, and uses traditional and complementary health care practices as appropriate.

- ▶ Utilizes technology to measure, record, and retrieve traveler and trip data.

- ▶ Incorporates technology to implement the nursing process, and enhance nursing practice (e.g., global disease surveillance systems).

- ▶ Uses evidence-based interventions and treatments specific to the diagnosis or travel-related problem.

- ▶ Participates, with traveler agreement, in assessing and assuring responsible use of interventions to minimize unwarranted or unwanted treatment and traveler suffering.

- ▶ Interprets surveillance data related to the plan and traveler health status.

- ▶ Applies appropriate knowledge of major travel-related risks and cultural diversity of the itinerary in implementing the plan of care.

- ▶ Facilitates utilization of systems, organizations, and community resources in the United States and at destination to implement the plan.

- ▶ Collaborates with healthcare providers from diverse backgrounds in the United States, and as needed, internationally, to implement and integrate the plan.

- ▶ Implements the plan in a timely manner in accordance with travel goals.

- ▶ Promotes the traveler's capacity for the optimal level of participation and problem solving.

▶ Documents implementation and any modifications, including changes or omissions, of the identified plan as appropriate.

Additional Competencies for the Graduate-Level Prepared Travel Health Nurse and the APRN

The graduate-level prepared travel health nurse or the advanced practice registered nurse:

▶ Uses principles and concepts of project or systems management.

▶ Fosters organizational systems that support implementation of the plan.

▶ Participates in the development of written policies and procedures for the clinical services and programs addressing travel health.

▶ Participates in the implementation of written policies and procedures for the clinical services and programs addressing travel health.

▶ Mentors other travel health nurses on appropriate implementation of plans.

▶ Synthesizes empirical evidence on risk behaviors, behavior change theories, epidemiology, health communication models, learning theories, motivational theories, and other related theories and frameworks when designing travel health education information and travel health promotion programs.

▶ Evaluates travel health information sources for accuracy, clarity, and readability to help travelers access quality health information.

▶ Incorporates new knowledge and strategies to initiate change in nursing care practices as travel health risks and interventions evolve or if desired outcomes are not achieved.

▶ Incorporates comparative effectiveness research recommendations into travel health education and travel health promotion strategies.

▶ Provides leadership to travel health nursing and other travel health professionals in planning evidence-based travel health promotion programs and services based upon current assessments, identification of population-specific and prioritized needs, identification of global health and safety risks, understanding of policy issues, and appropriate planning and evaluation strategies.

- ▶ Engages advocacy groups and travel alliances, as appropriate, in health education and health promotion activities.
- ▶ Modifies existing travel health education and travel health promotion programs based on feedback from participants, providers, health professionals, and other stakeholders.
- ▶ Designs solutions to internal and external barriers or challenges that may affect implementation of the plan.
- ▶ Advocates for needed resources for implementation of the plan with the traveler.
- ▶ Champions new and ongoing collaborative relationships to implement the plan.

Standard 5A. Coordination of Care

The travel health nurse coordinates care delivery.

Competencies

The travel health nurse:

▶ Organizes the components of the plan to maximize independence and health and safety during and after travel.

▶ Assists the traveler in identifying options for other health care services as indicated.

▶ Educates the traveler that travel health standards vary among countries and may differ from the U.S. standard of care (e.g., vaccine availability, vaccination schedules, medications).

▶ Communicates with the traveler and other parties as appropriate during transitions in care.

▶ Advocates for the delivery of timely, dignified, culturally competent, developmentally appropriate, and humane care by the interprofessional team.

▶ Coordinates delivery of supports and services as identified in the healthcare plan.

▶ Provides for the continuity of supports and services as identified in the healthcare plan.

▶ Documents the coordination of care and referrals.

▶ Educates colleagues regarding implementation of the plan.

▶ Applies best practices for coordination to attain effective travel health nursing care.

Additional Competencies for the Graduate-Level Prepared Travel Health Nurse and the APRN

The graduate-level prepared travel health nurse or the advanced practice registered nurse:

- ▶ Provides leadership in the coordination of interprofessional health care (U.S. and internationally prn) for integrated delivery of travel health care.

- ▶ Synthesizes data and information to prescribe necessary system and community support measures.

Standard 5B. Health Teaching and Health Promotion
The travel health nurse employs multiple strategies to promote health and safety during and after travel.

Competencies

The travel health nurse:

- ▶ Includes appropriate health education in the planning and implementation of programs and services for travelers, including, but not limited to:
  - ► Available resources in the United States and internationally;
  - ► Developmental needs;
  - ► Healthy lifestyle choices and behavior;
  - ► Health promotion, disease prevention, and risk-reduction strategies (e.g., selection of safer food and beverages, correct use of repellents); and
  - ► Multiple determinants of health (e.g., climate, zoonoses).
- ▶ Uses evidence-based health promotion and health teaching methods appropriate to the situation and the traveler's values, beliefs, health practices, developmental level, learning needs, readiness and ability to learn, language preferences, spirituality, culture, dates of travel, and socioeconomic status.
- ▶ Provides anticipatory guidance to the traveler to promote health and safety.
- ▶ Offers anticipatory guidance to the traveler to prevent or reduce the risk of travel-related and safety problems, both vaccine preventable and non-vaccine preventable.
- ▶ Counsels travelers with information about intended effects and potential adverse effects of proposed care plan (e.g., vaccine benefits, risk of anaphylaxis).
- ▶ Provides opportunities for feedback and evaluation of the effectiveness of the teaching strategies used.
- ▶ Uses appropriate, updated information technology to deliver health promotion and disease prevention information to the traveler in a variety of settings (e.g., health maps, CDC travel health applications).

- Incorporates an ecological perspective and knowledge of the multiple determinants of health to work effectively with diverse travel populations (e.g., seniors, college students, employees).

- Provides individual and group health teaching and health counseling for and with travelers.

- Evaluates health information resources, such as those available on the internet, within the area of practice for accuracy, readability, and comprehensibility.

- Assists travelers to access quality health information resources, such as those available on the internet.

- Serves as a primary resource to clinical staff and others regarding travel health information.

Additional Competencies for the Graduate-Level Prepared Travel Health Nurse and the APRN

The graduate-level prepared travel nurse or the advanced practice registered nurse:

- Synthesizes empirical evidence on risk behaviors, epidemiology, health communication models, and theories of behavioral change, learning, motivation, and other related theories and frameworks when designing health education information and health promotion programs.

- Incorporates comparative effectiveness research recommendations into travel health education and health promotion strategies.

- Provides leadership to nursing and other healthcare professionals in planning evidence-based travel health promotion programs and services based upon current assessments, identification of traveler-specific and prioritized needs, understanding of travel issues, and appropriate planning and evaluation strategies.

- Engages advocacy groups and consumer alliances, as appropriate, in travel health education and promotion activities.

- Modifies existing travel health education and promotion programs and policies based on feedback from participants, providers, health professionals, and other stakeholders.

Standard 6. Evaluation

The travel health nurse evaluates progress toward attainment of outcomes.

Competencies

The travel health nurse:

▶ Conducts a systematic, ongoing, and criterion-based evaluation of the outcomes in relation to the structures and processes prescribed by the pre-travel plan of care and indicated timeline.

▶ Evaluates, in partnership with the traveler and others, the effectiveness of the planned strategies, including complementary and alternative therapies, in relation to the traveler's responses and the attainment of the expected outcomes (e.g., no malaria infection, appropriate follow-up of a dog bite, etc.).

▶ Utilizes ongoing assessment data to identify gaps and redundancies in the travel health plan.

▶ Uses ongoing assessment data to revise travel health plans, interventions, and activities as needed for the benefit of the traveler and the communities to which they journey and return.

▶ Participates in assessing the responsible and appropriate use of interventions in order to minimize unwarranted or unwanted treatment, unnecessary costs, and traveler suffering.

▶ Documents the results of the evaluation.

Additional Competencies for the Graduate-Level Prepared Travel Health Nurse and the APRN

The graduate-level prepared travel nurse or the advanced practice registered nurse:

▶ Designs an evaluation plan with other travel health experts and with traveler representatives and other stakeholders that evaluates the accuracy of a travel health need.

▶ Proposes an evaluation plan with other travel health experts and with traveler representatives and other stakeholders that evaluates the effectiveness of the prevention or treatment plan.

- ▶ Collects data systematically, applying epidemiological and scientific methods to determine the effectiveness of travel health nursing interventions on policies, programs, and services.

- ▶ Aggregates the data from travel health outcomes to modify change in policies and procedures that support healthy travelers.

- ▶ Gathers data from travel health outcomes to promote travel health programs that support healthy travelers.

Standards of Professional Performance for Travel Health Nursing

Standard 7. Ethics

The travel health nurse practices ethically.

Competencies

The travel health nurse:

- ▶ Uses *The Code of Ethics for Nurses With Interpretive Statements* (ANA, 2015) to guide practice.

- ▶ Utilizes the *Code of Ethics for Travel Health Nurses* (ATHNA, 2017) to guide practice.

- ▶ Delivers care in a manner that preserves and protects traveler autonomy, dignity, rights, values, and beliefs.

- ▶ Recognizes the centrality of the traveler as a core member of the healthcare team.

- ▶ Upholds privacy and confidentiality of travelers and their data and information within legal and regulatory parameters.

- ▶ Assists travelers in self-determination and informed consent decision-making.

- ▶ Maintains a therapeutic and professional traveler–nurse relationship within appropriate professional role boundaries.

- ▶ Contributes to resolving ethical issues involving travelers, destination populations, colleagues, community groups, systems, and other stakeholders.

- ▶ Takes appropriate action regarding instances of illegal, unethical, or inappropriate behavior that can endanger or jeopardize the best interests of the traveler or the destination (e.g. human trafficking).

▶ Questions healthcare practice when necessary for safety and quality improvement.

▶ Advocates for equitable traveler care for all travel populations in all practice settings.

▶ Participates in inter-professional teams that address ethical risks, benefits, and outcomes.

▶ Provides information on the risks, benefits, and outcomes of healthcare regimens to allow informed decision-making by the traveler, including informed consent and informed refusal.

▶ Integrates caring, kindness and respect into nursing practice.

▶ Maintains competence through continued personal and professional development.

▶ Partners with multisector team members to address ethical risks, benefits, and outcomes of policies, programs, and services.

▶ Acts as a consultant to others to resolve ethical issues of travelers, destination populations, colleagues, or others.

▶ Provides leadership to the development and operation of an ethics committee in the clinical setting.

Standard 8. Culturally Congruent Practice

The travel health nurse practices in a manner that is congruent with cultural diversity and inclusion principles.

Competencies

The travel health nurse:

- ▶ Recognizes the impact of culture and cultural differences on the travel health encounter.
- ▶ Demonstrates respect, equity, and empathy in actions and inter-actions with all travelers including VFR travelers, immigrants, and refugees.
- ▶ Creates an inventory of one's own values, beliefs, and cultural heritage.
- ▶ Participates in periodic self-assessment of personal biases and reactions to travelers who have different backgrounds from the travel health nurse.
- ▶ Demonstrates knowledge of world geography, geo-political concerns, the health environment, and the sociocultural customs of a traveler's destination.
- ▶ Participates in lifelong learning, sensitivity training, and travel to understand cultural preferences, worldview, and decision-making processes of diverse travelers and destination countries.
- ▶ Applies knowledge of variations in health beliefs, practices, and com-munication patterns in travel health nursing practice.
- ▶ Considers the effects and impact of discrimination and oppression on vulnerable cultural groups (e.g., LGBTQ+ travelers, travelers with HIV, migrants, refugees).
- ▶ Contemplates the effects and impact of sex tourism, exploited hosts, voluntourism, romance tourism, ecotourism, and medical tourism on travelers and destination countries.
- ▶ Uses skills and tools that are appropriately vetted for the culture, literacy, and language of the population served (e.g., cultural ques-tionnaires, multilanguage CDC Vaccine Information Statements, IAC multilanguage educational handouts).

- ► Communicates with appropriate language and behaviors, including the use of medical interpreters and translators in accordance with traveler preferences.

- ► Recognizes the cultural variations of interactions, terms, and content. The nurse recognizes cultural and sub-cultural differences in personal space requirements, eye contact, time and punctuality, dress and body decoration, touch, food choices, religious impact on vaccine choices (e.g. porcine), and traditional medications and treatments (e.g., herbal supplements, cupping).

- ► Raises awareness among colleagues, travelers and the public of social, environmental, cultural and health issues caused by travel and tourism within destination communities.

- ► Respects traveler decisions based on age, gender, ethnicity, religion, education, occupation, socioeconomic status, and other related variants such as tradition, belief and family influence, and stage of acculturation.

- ► Supports policies that promote health and safety among culturally diverse, underserved, or underrepresented travelers as well as the communities to which they travel and return.

- ► Advocates for policies that promote health and safety, equity, veracity, and affordability among the travel and pharmaceutical industries.

- ► Promotes adherence to international principles of responsible and culturally sensitive travel (e.g., WHO, CDC, ISTM) among travelers and key travel health stakeholders.

- ► Promotes equal access to services, tests, interventions, health promotion programs, and enrollment in research, education, and other opportunities for travelers at home and internationally.

- ► Educates travel health colleagues and other professionals about cultural similarities and differences of travelers, families, groups, destination communities, and global populations.

- ► Speaks out against U.S. or international policies that discriminate against, oppress, or otherwise result in harm toward specific cultural groups.

Additional Competencies for the Graduate-Level Prepared Travel Health Nurse

The graduate-level prepared travel health nurse:

- ▶ Evaluates tools, instruments, and services provided to culturally diverse travel populations for effectiveness in assessing specific group and individual needs.

- ▶ Advances organizational travel health nursing policies, programs, services and practices that reflect respect, equity, and values for diversity, inclusion, and global wellness.

- ▶ Engages travelers, travel health nursing colleagues, key travel industry stakeholders, and others in designing and establishing internal and external cross-cultural partnerships through participation in international organizations that promote travel health including ISTM and ATHNA.

- ▶ Conducts research to improve pre- and post-travel healthcare access and healthcare outcomes for culturally diverse travelers (e.g., VFR travelers, immigrants, refugees).

- ▶ Participates in research to protect local destination communities from negative impacts of tourism and home communities from public health concerns.

- ▶ Develops strategies to protect local destination communities from negative impacts of tourism and home communities from public health concerns.

- ▶ Develops recruitment and retention strategies to achieve a multicultural workforce skilled in travel health including nurses fluent in multiple languages.

- ▶ Leads interprofessional teams to identify the cultural and language needs of travelers.

Additional Competencies for APRNs

In addition to the competencies of the registered nurse and the graduate-level prepared registered nurse, the advanced practice registered nurse:

▶ Promotes shared decision-making solutions in planning, prescribing, and evaluating processes when the traveler's cultural preferences and norms may create incompatibility with evidence-based practice (e.g. female genital mutilation).

Standard 9. Communication

The travel health nurse communicates effectively in a variety of formats in all areas of practice.

Competencies

The travel health nurse:

- ▶ Expresses ideas clearly and concisely.
- ▶ Disseminates information about travel health nursing decisions, plans, and recommendations for the domestic and international traveler via verbal and written communications and role play of common traveler situations.
- ▶ Communicates critical information to the traveler in all aspects of travel health to limit/avoid unfamiliarity with destinations, culture and health risks encountered in travel, and plans for appropriate pre- and post-travel care.
- ▶ Encourages direct and open discussions about important issues with travelers, colleagues, and other travel health stakeholders.
- ▶ Practices communication skills to promote healthy relationships between nurses and travelers.
- ▶ Uses communication skills to provide a context for open discussion of traveler experiences.
- ▶ Utilizes communication skills to improve traveler outcomes in question and answer dialogue.
- ▶ Accommodates for different styles of communication used by travelers and healthcare providers.
- ▶ Communicates with travelers and healthcare providers regarding traveler care and the nurse's role in the provision of that care.
- ▶ Documents clearly and concisely, using terminology understood by national and international colleagues.
- ▶ Communicates in accordance with all applicable regulations concerning confidentiality and traveler privacy (e.g., HIPAA, institutional guidelines).
- ▶ Evaluates verbal and written communication format preferences of travelers and colleagues (e.g., language, literacy level).

- Assesses his or her own communication skills, travel health literacy, resources, and preferences in encounters with travelers and interprofessional team colleagues.

- Seeks continuous improvement of communication and conflict resolution skills through self-assessment, peer review, and training.

- Conveys information to travelers, the interprofessional team, and others in communication formats that promote accuracy and adherence to U.S. standards of travel health care (e.g., CDC, ACIP).

- Questions the rationale supporting care processes and decisions when they do not appear to be in the best interest of the traveler.

- Discloses observations or concerns related to travel health hazards and errors in care or the practice environment to the appropriate management level and appropriate public health officials.

- Maintains communication with other providers to minimize or eliminate potential error risks associated with transfers and transitions in travel healthcare delivery.

- Contributes his or her own professional perspective in discussions with the interprofessional team.

- Documents communications to promote accountability in practice.

- Follows communication policies and procedures to ensure compliance with regulatory requirements.

- Assimilates health literacy principles into travel health communications with individuals, families, groups, and communities.

Additional Competencies for the Graduate-Level Prepared Travel Health Nurse and the APRN

The graduate-level prepared travel health nurse or advanced practice registered nurse:

- Integrates advanced health literacy principles into travel health communications with individuals, families, groups, and communities.

- Demonstrates system-levels and global approach critical thinking and communication skills in travel health patient and colleague encounters.

▶ Thinks critically about evidence-based practice and applies or communicates the information to improve the standards of travel health nursing.

▶ Contributes knowledge from the humanities and other disciplines to communications in travel health nursing.

▶ Incorporates research findings to enhance travel health nursing patient encounters and practice methods.

▶ Includes research findings to enhance traveler health and safety outcomes.

▶ Creates fresh evidence-based communication approaches and techniques, paying attention to research findings, core theory, and experience from travel health practice for the benefit of the traveler, the destination, and the community to which the traveler returns.

▶ Mentors other colleagues in presentation and dissemination of travel health information to patients and colleagues.

▶ Assumes a leadership role in travel health nursing, shaping or fashioning environments that promote healthy communication nationally and internationally with colleagues, other health professionals, and the public.

Standard 10. Collaboration

The travel health nurse collaborates with the traveler and others in the conduct of nursing practice.

Competencies

The travel health nurse:

▶ Partners with other health professionals to effect change and produce positive outcomes through the sharing of knowledge of the traveler and the itinerary.

▶ Participates in building consensus or resolving conflict in the context of traveler care.

▶ Applies group process and negotiation techniques with travelers and colleagues.

▶ Adheres to the standards and applicable codes of conduct that govern behavior among peers and colleagues to create a work environment that promotes cooperation, respect, and trust.

▶ Engages in teamwork and the team-building process.

▶ Invites the contribution of the traveler and team members to achieve optimal outcomes.

▶ Documents plan-of-care communications, rationales for plan-of-care changes and collaborative discussions to improve traveler outcomes.

Additional Competencies for the Graduate-Level Prepared Travel Health Nurse and the APRN

The graduate-level prepared travel health nurse and the advanced practice registered nurse:

▶ Partners with other disciplines to enhance traveler outcomes through interprofessional activities, such as education, consultation, management, technological development, or research opportunities.

▶ Serves as a leader in establishing, improving, and sustaining collaborative relationships to achieve safe, quality traveler care.

Standard 11. Leadership
The travel health nurse leads within the professional practice setting and the profession.

Competencies

The travel health nurse:

- ▶ Oversees the nursing care given by ancillary personnel in accordance with state regulations while retaining accountability for the quality of care given to the traveler.

- ▶ Incorporates the vision and goals of the travel health organization when planning and implementing care and measuring progress of an individual traveler.

- ▶ Demonstrates a commitment to continuous, lifelong learning and education for self and others.

- ▶ Mentors colleagues for the advancement of travel health nursing practice, the nursing profession, and quality travel health care.

- ▶ Treats colleagues with respect, trust, and dignity.

- ▶ Uses communication and conflict resolution skills.

- ▶ Participates in travel health societies, travel health nursing, and other professional organizations.

- ▶ Communicates effectively with the traveler and colleagues.

- ▶ Seeks ways to advance travel health nursing autonomy and accountability.

- ▶ Participates in efforts to influence healthcare policy involving travelers and the travel health profession.

- ▶ Provides input into the budget for nursing and travel health services.

- ▶ Shares in the design of new nurse's offices, health rooms, or travel health clinics.

Additional Competencies for the Graduate-Level Prepared Travel Health Nurse and the APRN

The graduate-level prepared travel health nurse or advanced practice registered nurse:

▶ Serves in leadership roles in professional organizations and committees at local, state, national, and international levels.

▶ Influences decision-making authorities to improve the professional practice environment and traveler health outcomes via research, publication, and teaching.

▶ Provides direction to enhance the effectiveness of the interprofessional travel health team.

▶ Promotes travel health advanced nursing practice and role development by interpreting its role for travelers and others.

▶ Models expert practice to interprofessional team members and travelers.

▶ Mentors colleagues in the acquisition of clinical knowledge, skills, abilities, and decision-making.

▶ Shapes direction of the specialty by actively engaging in such initiatives as development of standards, competencies, role definitions, position statements, and clinical guidelines.

▶ Analyzes the interactions of systems and their influence on the practice of travel health nursing.

▶ Incorporates a global focus when examining the practice of travel health nursing.

▶ Advocates for funding of travel health services.

Standard 12. Education

The travel health nurse attains knowledge and competence that reflects current travel health nursing practice and incorporates emerging trends.

Competencies

The travel health nurse:

▶ Participates in ongoing educational activities related to appropriate knowledge bases and professional issues.

▶ Demonstrates a commitment to lifelong learning through self-reflection and inquiry to address learning and personal growth needs.

▶ Acquires knowledge and skills appropriate to the role, travel populations served, or setting.

▶ Seeks formal education and experiential learning opportunities to develop and maintain clinical and professional knowledge, skills, abilities, and judgment in clinical practice or role performance.

▶ Identifies learning needs based on travel health nursing knowledge, the various roles the travel health nurse may assume, the changing needs of the traveler, and changes in global health and safety epidemiology, policies, and regulations.

▶ Uses current healthcare research findings and other evidence to expand clinical knowledge, skills, abilities, and judgment, to enhance travel health nursing performance, and to increase knowledge of professional issues.

▶ Shares educational findings, experiences, and ideas with peers to promote a current standard of practice.

▶ Participates in formal or informal consultations with travel health experts to address issues in nursing practice as an application of education and a knowledge base.

▶ Communicates educational findings, experiences, and ideas with peers nationally and internationally.

▶ Contributes to a work environment conducive to the education of travel health professionals.

▶ Maintains professional records that provide evidence of competence and lifelong learning.

Additional Competencies for the Graduate-Level Prepared Travel Health Nurse and the APRN

The graduate-level prepared travel health nurse or the advanced practice registered nurse:

▶ Provides professional education to other travel health nurses and other professionals including other nursing, medical, pharmacy, public health, veterinary medicine, mental health, corporate executives, student health administrators, military, and risk management personnel as well as many others.

▶ Leads the development of travel health education and educational programming.

▶ Acts as a consultant to other health care providers and educational groups on travel health nursing education.

▶ Mentors travel health nursing students and those early in their careers.

Standard 13. Evidence-Based Practice and Research

The travel health nurse integrates evidence and research findings into practice.

Competencies

The travel health nurse:

- ▶ Engages in ongoing review and evaluation of the literature relevant to travel health nursing.
- ▶ Critically evaluates research using criteria for scientific merit including appropriate design, data collection and analysis, and ethical standards.
- ▶ Utilizes current evidence-based travel health knowledge, including research findings, to guide practice.
- ▶ Identifies clinical concerns related to the practice of travel health nursing, searching for solutions.
- ▶ Synthesizes and appraises the best available travel health evidence to recommend practice changes.
- ▶ Applies principles of implementation science to maintain and sustain practice changes that benefit the health of the traveler, the destination(s), and the community to which the traveler returns.
- ▶ Participates, as appropriate to educational level and position, in the formulation of evidence-based practice through research.
- ▶ Shares personal or third-party research findings with colleagues and peers, patients, and other relevant stakeholders.
- ▶ Evaluates the outcomes of evidence-based interventions on an ongoing basis.
- ▶ Acts as a champion of scientific inquiry, generating new knowledge and integrating best available evidence into practice of travel health nursing.

Additional Competencies for the Graduate-Level Prepared Travel Health Nurse and the APRN

The graduate-level prepared travel health nurse or the advanced practice registered nurse:

▶ Contributes to nursing knowledge by conducting or synthesizing research and other evidence that discovers, examines, and evaluates current practice, knowledge, theories, criteria, and creative approaches to improve travel health outcomes.

▶ Promotes a climate of research and clinical inquiry.

▶ Contributes to inter-professional practice by supporting, conducting, and synthesizing travel health and travel health nursing research and evidence-based practice.

▶ Implements research activities to align with the goals of regulatory travel health organizations and recognized experts of travel health.

▶ Ensures that research undergoes review by an institutional review board in accordance with national guidelines and legal and ethical stipulations.

▶ Demonstrates that research is consistent with improved patient outcomes as they relate to travel health.

▶ Disseminates research findings to relevant entities, such as the ISTM, ATHNA, and AAOHN, through presentations, publications, consultation, blogs and other social media outlets, and journal clubs.

▶ Disseminates research, evidence-based practice, and quality improvement findings through presentations, publication, and consultation.

▶ Incorporates research findings and evidenced-based recommendations into policies, procedures, and patient care guidelines across organizations locally, nationally, and internationally.

▶ Initiates research opportunities for nursing staff, mentoring less experienced travel health nurses participating in research.

▶ Encourages nursing staff to participate in learning opportunities, quality assurance activities, and research initiatives to enhance the delivery of travel health nursing services and promote travel health nursing practice.

▶ Advocates for resources for nurses to engage in all aspects of the research process and further scientific inquiry.

► Advances the science of nursing professional development through mentoring and serving as a travel health nursing resource to colleagues and peers.

► Recognizes the contributions of nurse scientists and researchers within organizations and professional groups.

Standard 14. Quality of Practice

The travel health nurse contributes to quality nursing practice.

Competencies

The travel health nurse:

▶ Participates in clinical inquiry through quality improvement activities.

▶ Demonstrates quality by documenting the application of the nursing process in a responsible, accountable, and ethical manner.

▶ Uses creativity and innovation to enhance travel health care (e.g., group counseling, use of travel health apps, role play, tele-health, point of care diagnostics).

▶ Participates in quality improvement in a systematic, formal approach to the analysis of practice performance and efforts to improve performance in travel health nursing.

▶ Identifies aspects of pre-, intransit, and post-travel practice important for quality monitoring (e.g., compliance with HIPAA, completion of multi-dose vaccine series, post-trip monitoring for fever).

▶ Uses indicators to monitor quality, safety, and effectiveness of travel health nursing practice (e.g., post vaccination adverse events, epinephrine auto-injector demonstration).

▶ Collects data to monitor quality and effectiveness of travel health nursing practice (e.g., post-travel fever surveys, recall surveys of pre-travel health counseling).

▶ Describes the structure, function, and authority of the organizational units within local, state, federal agencies, and WHO, and their impact on travel health nursing practice.

▶ Educates the traveler on the development and application of relevant laws, regulations, and policies (e.g. access to yellow fever vaccine).

▶ Supports all relevant travel health policies, programs, and resources (e.g., ACIP, WHO, institutional).

▶ Completes monitoring and inspection activities for regulated entities (e.g. VFC audits).

- Collects specific information about situations that are reported to travel health officials to inform policy decisions (e.g., VAERS, reportable diseases).

- Monitors changes in international travel health related laws, policies, and regulations (e.g., yellow fever vaccination requirement, requirements for the Hajj, etc.).

- Assists with addressing noncompliance with guidelines, laws, regulations, and policies.

- Contributes to the inter-professional team to implement travel health regulatory requirements.

- Analyzes national and international quality data to identify opportunities for improving travel health nursing practice during the pre-, intransit, and post-travel encounter.

- Evaluates policies, procedures, activities, recommendations and guidelines to improve the quality of travel health nursing practice (e.g. evaluates pre-travel and post-travel assessment tools to concur with annual ACIP vaccination recommendations).

- Participates in efforts to minimize immunization and additional visit costs and unnecessary vaccination duplication.

- Identifies travel health nursing concerns such as no-show appointments and expired or wasted vaccines, which occur in day-to-day work routines in order to correct process inefficiencies.

- Analyzes factors related to quality, safety and travel health nursing effectiveness (e.g., time allowance for appointments, health counseling comprehension).

- Analyzes organizational systems for barriers to quality travel health outcomes.

- Implements processes to remove or weaken barriers within organizational systems.

- Obtains and maintains professional certification if it is available in the area of expertise.

Additional Competencies for the Graduate-Level Prepared Travel Health Nurse and the APRN

The graduate-level prepared travel health nurse or the advanced practice registered nurse:

▶ Provides advanced leadership in the design and implementation of quality improvements through education, research, and publication on travel health topics.

▶ Designs innovations to effect change in travel health nursing practice and travel health practice overall and improve traveler health and safety outcomes.

▶ Evaluates the practice environment and quality of travel health nursing care rendered in relation to existing evidence.

▶ Obtains travel health histories and assesses, diagnoses, prescribes, and treats within scope of practice for both acute and chronic illnesses that may impact the traveler on the journey and upon return home.

▶ Investigates effects of traveler's health and behaviors on the destination and effects of destination exposures on the community to which the traveler returns.

▶ Offers referrals for specialized care as indicated for pre- and post-travel at home and internationally.

▶ Discusses transcultural knowledge about health, safety, and environmental factors related to nursing perspectives, the individual traveler, and the destination(s).

▶ Completes data analysis and report generation for travel health officials and others as required by law, regulations, and policies.

▶ Identifies opportunities for the generation and use of travel health research and evidence.

▶ Uses the results of quality improvement to initiate changes in travel health nursing practices and the healthcare delivery system.

▶ Provides leadership in the design and implementation of quality improvements.

▶ Evaluates the practice environment and quality of travel health nursing care rendered in relation to existing evidence.

▶ Identifies opportunities for the generation and use of research and evidence.

▶ Uses the results of quality improvement to initiate changes in travel health nursing practices and the healthcare delivery system.

Standard 15. Professional Practice Evaluation

The travel health nurse evaluates his or her own nursing practice and that of others.

Competencies

The travel health nurse:

- ► Engages in self-evaluation of practice on a regular basis, identifying areas of strength as well as areas in which professional growth would be beneficial.

- ► Obtains informal and formal feedback regarding his or her own practice from travelers, peers, professional colleagues, and others.

- ► Participates in peer review and audit procedures as appropriate.

- ► Takes action to achieve goals identified during the evaluation process.

- ► Provides the evidence for practice decisions and actions as part of the informal and formal evaluation processes.

- ► Interacts with peers and colleagues to enhance his or her professional nursing practice or role performance.

- ► Conveys to peers formal or informal constructive feedback regarding his or her practice or role performance.

- ► Engages in a formal process seeking feedback regarding his or her practice from travelers, peers, professional colleagues, and others.

Additional Competencies for the Graduate-Level Prepared Travel Health Nurse and the APRN

The graduate-level prepared travel health nurse and the advanced practice registered nurse:

- ► Audits the professional practice evaluation analyses to recommend or make changes including policy, procedure, or service revision, as appropriate.

- ► Ascertains follow up of audit finding recommendations to improve quality of travel health nursing.

Standard 16. Resource Utilization

The travel health nurse uses appropriate resources to plan, provide, and sustain evidence-based nursing services that are safe, effective, and financially responsible.

Competencies

The travel health nurse:

- ▶ Identifies traveler needs, potential for harm, complexity of the task, and desired outcomes when considering resource allocation.
- ▶ Delegates elements of care to appropriate healthcare workers in accordance with any applicable legal or policy parameters or principles.
- ▶ Identifies evidence-based practice when evaluating resources.
- ▶ Advocates for resources, including technology, that enhance travel health nursing practice and the traveler experience.
- ▶ Modifies practice when necessary to promote positive interaction between travelers, care providers, and technology.
- ▶ Assists the traveler in identifying and securing appropriate services to address needs across the healthcare continuum.
- ▶ Assists the traveler in factoring costs, risks, and benefits in decisions about treatment and care.
- ▶ Utilizes organizational and community resources to formulate inter-professional plans of care.
- ▶ Formulates innovative solutions for traveler care problems that effectively utilize resources in the United States, and as needed, internationally, to maintain quality.
- ▶ Integrates tele-health and mobile health technologies into practice to promote positive interactions between travelers, travel health nurse, and other care providers.
- ▶ Addresses discriminatory healthcare practices and the impact on resource allocation.

Additional Competencies for the Graduate-Level Prepared Travel Health Nurse and the APRN

The graduate-level prepared travel health nurse and the advanced practice registered nurse:

▶ Designs evaluation strategies that demonstrate cost-effectiveness, cost-benefit, and efficiency factors associated with travel health nursing practice.

Standard 17. Environmental Health

The travel health nurse practices in an environmentally safe and healthy manner.

Competencies

The travel health nurse:

- ▶ Maintains knowledge of environmental health concepts, such as implementation of environmental health strategies.

- ▶ Promotes a travel health practice environment that reduces environmental health risks for workers and travelers.

- ▶ Assesses the practice environment for factors such as sound, odor, noise, and light that threaten health.

- ▶ Advocates for the judicious and appropriate use of products in travel health care as well as disposal of products and packaging.

- ▶ Communicates information about environmental health risks and exposure reduction strategies to travelers, colleagues, and communities.

- ▶ Utilizes scientific evidence to determine if a product or treatment is an environmental threat to the traveler, the destination or the community to which the traveler returns (e.g. sunscreen use in bioluminescent bays).

- ▶ Participates in developing strategies to promote healthy travelers and communities in the United States and internationally.

- ▶ Disposes of medical waste from the travel health encounter (e.g., syringes, blood contaminated dressings) in accordance with local laws and environmental regulations.

- ▶ Counsels travelers to be thoughtful of natural resources when traveling (e.g., appropriate waste disposal, avoidance of excessive water use in showers or baths, leaving the environment undisturbed, averting purchase of souvenirs containing animal products such as shells or skins).

Additional Competencies for the Graduate-Level Prepared Travel Health Nurse and the APRN

The graduate-level prepared travel health nurse and the advanced practice registered nurse:

▶ Creates partnerships that promote global sustainable environmental health policies and conditions (e.g., CDC, WHO, RCN, Faculty of Travel Medicine, Royal College of Physicians and Surgeons of Glasgow).

▶ Analyzes the impact of social, political, and economic influences on the environment and human health exposures.

▶ Critically evaluates the manner in which environmental health issues are presented by the media.

▶ Advocates for implementation of environmental principles for travel health nursing practice.

▶ Supports nurses in advocating for and implementing environmental principles in travel health nursing practice.

Glossary

ACIP. The Advisory Committee on Immunization Practices is a CDC agency comprised of medical and public health experts who make recommendations for the use of vaccines to protect the health of the United States population. (ACIP https://www.cdc.gov/vaccines/acip/index.html)

Advanced practice registered nurse (APRN). A nurse who has completed an accredited graduate-level education program preparing her or him for the role of certified nurse practitioner, certified nurse anesthetist, certified nurse-midwife or clinical nurse specialist; has passed a national certification examination that measures the APRN role and population-focused competencies; maintains continued competence as evidenced by recertification; and is licensed to practice as an APRN. (Adapted from APRN JDG, 2008)

American Association of Occupational Health Nurses (AAOHN). The AAOHN is the professional association of licensed nurses engaged in the practice of occupation and environmental health nursing. (AAOHN http://aaohn.org/)

American College Health Association (ACHA). This association serves as the principal leadership organization for advancing the health of college students and campus communities through advocacy, education, and research. (ACHA https://www.acha.org/)

American Nurses Association (ANA). The American Nurses Association, a professional organization which advances and protects the profession of nursing.

American Society of Tropical Medicine and Hygiene (ASTMH). The largest international scientific organization of experts dedicated to reducing the worldwide burden of tropical infectious diseases and improving global health. ASTMH offers qualifying clinicians the CTropMed® credential. (ASTMH https://www.astmh.org/)

American Travel Health Nurses Association (ATHNA). The professional organization of travel health nurses promoting the health of travelers and their communities through evidence-based practice, research, and advocacy. (ATHNA, 2017)

Antimicrobial resistance. When microorganisms such as bacteria, viruses, fungi, and parasites change in ways that render the medications used to cure the infections they cause ineffective.

Assessment. A systematic, dynamic process by which the registered nurse, through interaction with the patient, family, groups, communities, populations, and healthcare providers, collects and analyzes data. Assessment is the initial step in the nursing process and may include the following dimensions: physical, psychological, sociocultural, spiritual, cognitive, functional abilities, developmental, economic, and lifestyle.

CE. Continuing education. Education provided for adults after they have left the formal education system, consisting typically of short or part-time courses.

Centers for Disease Control and Prevention (CDC). The federal agency that conducts and supports health promotion, prevention, and preparedness activities in the United States, with the goal of improving overall public health. The Travel Health Branch provides official U.S. government health recommendations for traveling for both providers and travelers. The branch also publishes the CDC "Yellow Book," *Health Information for International Travel* and posts Travel Health Notices regarding global outbreaks. (CDC https://wwwnc.cdc.gov/travel)

Chemoprophylaxis. The administration of a medication for the purpose of preventing disease or infection; also refers to the use of drugs before, during and after travel to prevent malaria, functional abilities, developmental, economic and lifestyle. (https://www.merriam-webster.com/dictionary/chemoprophylaxis)

Collaboration. A professional partnership grounded in a reciprocal and respectful recognition and acceptance of: each partner's unique expertise, power and sphere of influence and responsibilities; the commonality of goals; the mutual safeguarding of the legitimate interest of each party; and the advantages of such a relationship.

Conceptual framework. A theoretical structure or "network" of assumptions, principles, and rules that holds together the ideas comprising a broad concept.

CTH®. Certificate of Travel Health; refers to the interdisciplinary, international certificate awarded to health professionals who pass the ISTM CTH examination. (ISTM www.istm.org)

Cultural competence. A set of congruent behaviors, attitudes and policies that come together in a system or agency or among professionals and enables the system, agency or professionals to work effectively in cross-cultural settings.

Diagnosis. A clinical judgment about the healthcare consumer's response to actual or potential health conditions or needs. It is the second step in the nursing process and the basis for creating a plan with expected outcomes. The diagnosis provides the basis for determination of a plan to achieve expected outcomes. Registered nurses utilize nursing and medical diagnoses depending on educational and clinical preparation and legal authority.

Disinsection. The use of insecticides on international flights and in other closed spaces for insect and disease control; Pesticide applications, as may be mandated by certain countries to airplanes before, during, or after passenger transport. (U.S. Department of Transportation https://www.transportation.gov/airconsumer/spray)

Ecological model. A model of health that emphasizes the linkages and relationships among multiple factors affecting health. This approach focuses on both population-level and individual-level determinants of health and interventions. (ACHA https://www.acha.org/HealthyCampus/HealthyCampus/Ecological_Model.aspx)

Ectoparasites. A diverse group of organisms that infest the skin of humans and other animals. (Science Direct https://www.sciencedirect.com/topics/medicine-and-dentistry/ectoparasite)

Fitness-to-Travel examinations. This is a pre-travel health exam required by an employer or travel tour group to ensure that an employee or tour participant is physically and psychologically able to participate in a particular journey, often one requiring air travel or physical exertion.

Emergent diseases. Infections that have recently appeared within a population or those whose incidence or geographic range is rapidly increasing or threatens to increase in the near future (e.g., Zika, COVID-19). (Baylor College of Medicine https://www.bcm.edu/departments/molecular-virology-and-microbiology/emerging-infections-and-biodefense/emerging-infectious-diseases)

Emporiatrics. An older, alternative name for the specialty branch of medicine that deals with the prevention and management of health problems of international travelers. (Sushma, 2012)

Environmental health. Aspects of human health including quality of life, that are determined by physical, chemical, biological, social, and psychological problems in the environment. It also refers to the theory and practice of assessing, correcting, controlling, and preventing those factors in the environment that can potentially affect adversely the health of present and future generations.

Evidenced-Based practice. A scholarly and systematic problem-solving paradigm that results in the delivery of high-quality healthcare.

FGM. Female genital mutilation. (WHO https://www.who.int/news-room/fact-sheets/detail/female-genital-mutilation)

GeoSentinel. A global surveillance network for monitoring global disease among travelers. In 2018 it consists of 70 travel and tropical medicine centers situated in 31 countries across 6 continents. GeoSentinel was founded in 1995 by the International Society of Travel Medicine (ISTM) and is supported by ISTM the US Centers for Disease Control and Prevention and the Public Health Agency of Canada. (Journal of Travel Medicine https://academic.oup.com/jtm/article/25/1/tay139/5227422)

Global TravEpiNet. A national network of clinics across the United States that aims to improve the health of those who travel internationally. GTEN has created a series of web-based travel tools to improve the pre-travel health care of high-risk travelers. These tools are based on CDC recommendations. (CDC https://wwwnc.cdc.gov/travel/page/gten)

Graduate-level prepared specialty nurse. A registered nurse prepared at the master's or doctoral level who has advanced knowledge, skills, abilities, and judgment associated with one or more nursing specialties and is functioning in an advanced level as designated by elements of her or his position. (ANA, 2015)

Holistic. Characterized by the treatment of the whole person, taking into account mental and social factors, rather than just the symptoms of a disease; evidenced-based practice. A scholarly and systematic problem-solving paradigm that results in the delivery of high-quality healthcare.

IAC. The Immunization Action Coalition is the premier non-profit organization that provides U.S. health professionals with immunization information and education. (IAC http://www.immunize.org/)

IAMAT. The International Association for Medical Assistance to Travellers provides different resources for international travelers seeking health care during travel. (IAMAT https://www.iamat.org/)

ICVP. The *International Certificate of Vaccination or Prophylaxis,* also known as the "Yellow Card," is the WHO required documentation for yellow fever immunization. (CDC https://wwwnc.cdc.gov/travel)

IHR. International Health Regulations is a WHO international legal instrument that is binding on 196 countries across the globe, including all WHO member states. The purpose and scope of the IHR (2005) are "to prevent, protect against, control and provide a public health response to the international spread of disease in ways that are commensurate with and restricted to public health risks, and which avoid unnecessary interference with international trade." (WHO https://www.who.int/ihr/publications/9789241580496/en)

International Society of Travel Medicine (ISTM). An international organization comprised of health providers and others committed to the health and safety of global travelers. ISTM publishes the *Journal of Travel Medicine* and administers the CTH examination. (ISTM www.istm.org)

Intransit travel encounter. Refers to a travel health nursing encounter that occurs while the traveler is in transit; typically, this might be a phone call or email contact during a trip to address a health concern or issue. (ATHNA, 2017)

ISTM Body of Knowledge. A guide developed by ISTM for the professional development of any individual practicing travel medicine. International in focus, it can be used as one resource to help shape curricula and training programs in travel medicine. It does not address specific national standards of travel health care or different professional standards for physicians, nurses, pharmacists, and others. (ISTM www.istm.org)

Jerusalem Syndrome. An acute psychotic episode in travelers presenting with associated with religious delusions or obsessions. (Jewish Virtual Library https://www.jewishvirtuallibrary.org/the-jerusalem-syndrome)

Kumbh Mela. A mass Hindu pilgrimage of faith where Hindus gather to bathe in a holy river. It is the largest faith gathering in the world with millions of attendees and usually last 4 to 6 weeks in various locations in India. (Kumbh Mela https://kumbh.gov.in/en/about-kumbh)

NGO. A non-governmental organization is any non-profit, voluntary citizens' group which is organized on a local, national, or international level. Doctors Without Borders and the International Rescue Committee are two NGOs often associated with travel health issues. (NGO http://www.ngo.org/ngoinfo/define.html)

Nursing. The protection, promotion and optimization of health and abilities; prevention of illness and injury, facilitation of healing, alleviation of suffering through the diagnosis and treatment of human response, and advocacy in the care of individuals, families, communities and populations. (ANA, 2015)

Nursing practice. The collective professional activities of nurses characterized by the interrelations of human responses, theory application, nursing actions, and outcomes. (ANA, 2015)

Nursing process. A critical thinking model used by nurses that comprises the integration of the singular, concurrent actions by these six components: assessment, diagnosis, identification of outcomes, planning, implementation, and evaluation. (ANA, 2015)

Outbreaks. WHO defines these as the occurrence of cases of disease in excess of what would normally be expected in a defined community, geographical area, or season. (WHO http://www.searo.who.int/topics/disease_outbreaks/en)

Outcomes. Long-term objectives that define optimal, measurable future levels of health status, maximum acceptable levels of disease, injury or dysfunction, or prevalence of risk factors.

Planetary health. The integrative effort of multiple disciplines working locally, nationally, and globally to attain optimal health for people, animal, and the environment. Together, the three make up the "One Health" triad, and the health of each is inextricably connected to the others in the triad. (Rockefeller Foundation https://www.rockefellerfoundation.org/report/planetary-health-landscape-concept-action/).

Post-travel encounter. A clinical visit designed to evaluate and manage adverse health and safety outcomes of international travel. (ATHNA www.athna.org)

PPM. Personal protective measures: refers to techniques used to prevent insect bites, such as the use of long sleeve clothing, repellents, and bed-netting. (NCIB https://www.ncbi.nlm.nih.gov/pmc/articles/PMC2600214)

Pre-travel encounter. A clinical visit that focuses on the prevention of health and safety risks of a particular journey. While vaccinations are often included in this encounter, the travel health nurse focuses on health education and counseling. (ATHNA, 2017)

Principles of responsible travel. Guidelines for responsible tourism which minimize the negative social, economic, and environmental impacts, generates greater economic benefits for local people and enhances the well-being of host communities. These are principles of social and economic justice that exert full respect toward the travel environment and its cultures, and serve to foster a positive interaction between the tourist industry, the local communities, and the travelers. (Urban Land https://urbanland.uli.org/industry-sectors/ten-principles-responsible-tourism)

ProMed-mail. The Program for Monitoring Emerging Diseases is the International Society of Infectious Diseases internet-based reporting system dedicated to rapid global dissemination of information on outbreaks of infectious diseases and acute exposures to toxins that affect human health. (https://www.promedmail.org/aboutus/)

Quality. The degree to which health services for patients, families, groups, communities or populations increase the likelihood of desired outcomes and are consistent with current professional knowledge.

Quality improvement. Quality improvement is a systematic approach to continuous actions that lead to measurable improved outcomes. (ANA, 2015)

RCN. The Royal College of Nursing in the United Kingdom.

Recommended vaccinations. Immunizations that are designed to protect the traveler from vaccine-preventable diseases found at a particular destination (e.g., Japanese encephalitis, cholera, etc.; MedicineNet https://www.medicinenet.com/do_you_need_vaccinations_before_traveling_abroad/views.htm)

Required vaccinations. Immunizations mandated by order of WHO which are required to cross an international border (e.g., yellow fever vaccination for entry to Ghana; MedicineNet https://www.medicinenet.com/do_you_need_vaccinations_before_traveling_abroad/views.htm)

Routine vaccinations. Immunizations, recommended and updated yearly by the ACIP for U.S. infants, adolescents and adults (e.g., MMR, influenza, hepatitis B, etc.; ACIP www.acip.org)

Scope of nursing practice. The description of the what, when, where, who, how, when, and why of nursing practice that addresses the range of nursing practice activities common to all registered nurses. When considered in conjunction with the *Standards of Professional Nursing Practice* and the *Code of Ethics for Nurses*, comprehensively describes the competent level of nursing common to all registered nurses. (ANA, 2015)

Self-treatment. Treatment of oneself without professional supervision to alleviate an illness or condition; often travelers are provided with medications in the event they develop traveler's diarrhea or acute mountain sickness. (Shoreland https://tripprep.com/library/travelers-diarrhea/traveler-summary)

Spelunking. Caving.

Stakeholder. A person or organization that has an interest in what the travel health entity does.

Standards. Authoritative statements defined and promoted by the profession by which the quality of practice, service or education can be evaluated. (ANA, 2015)

Standards of practice. Describe a competent level of nursing care as demonstrated by the nursing process. See also: Nursing process. (ANA, 2015)

Standards of professional nursing practice. Authoritative statements of the duties that all registered nurses, regardless of role, population, or specialty, are expected to perform competently. (ANA, 2015)

Standards of professional performance. Describe a competent level of behavior in the professional role. (ANA, 2015)

Travax. A widely used commercial subscription software program that provides healthcare professionals with travel information and technology platforms to protect travelers. (Shoreland www.Shoreland.com)

Travel advisories and alerts. Updated country specific safety and security information published by the U.S. Department of State at https://travel.state.gov/content/travel/en/traveladvisories/traveladvisories.html/. There are four levels of alerts including Level 4: Do not travel. (U.S. State Dept.)

Travel Care. A commercial subscription software program that provides healthcare professionals with travel information and technology platforms to protect travelers. (Travel Care www.travelcare.com)

Travel health notices. Three levels of official U.S. government health recommendations for traveling published at https://wwwnc.cdc.gov/travel/notices. As provided by the CDC, these advisories are Level 1-Watch, Level 2-Alert, and Level 3-Warning during which all nonessential travel should be avoided to a particular country or region. (CDC)

Travel health nurse. A professional nurse who focuses on the health and safety of travelers through continuous surveillance and assessment of the multiple determinants of health with the intent to promote health and wellness, prevent disease, disability, and premature death before, during, and after travel. (ATHNA, 2017)

Travel health nursing. The specialized practice of professional nursing that advances the well-being of travelers. This specialty focuses on the health and safety of travelers through continuous surveillance and assessment of the multiple determinants of health with the intent to promote health and wellness, prevent disease, disability, and premature death.

Traveler. Defined as a person who is journeying from one destination (may be home environment) to another. Subcategories include but are not limited to (ATHNA, 2017):

- Air cruisers—persons traveling as a luxury group in one plane making multiple stops around the world on a prepaid, often very expensive itinerary
- Armed conflict regions (military, journalists, medics)
- Backpackers—a form of low-cost, independent travel; associated with a traveler carrying their belongings in a backpack
- Bucket list—lifelong "wish list" travel destinations or experiences
- Business traveler
  - Short-term—usually less than two-week duration
  - Frequent travelers—multiple returns to a specific country or region, or multiple trips within a month or year to different destinations
  - Ex-pat/long-term assignments—temporary residence of three or more months, may include family relocation
  - Flex-pat—newer, alternative employer arrangement that involves an employee making frequent return visits to same location, often for durations of two to six weeks with no relocation of family
- Ecotourists—tourism directed toward exotic, often threatened, natural environments, especially to support conservation efforts and observe wildlife
- Educational traveler
  - Students study abroad for durations of one week to multiple years
  - Conference attendees
  - Seniors traveling as part of course or another educational objective
- Families with children of all ages
- FGM travelers—families seeking *female* genital mutilation of relatives abroad
- High altitude traveler—person traveling to altitudes typically above 10,000 feet, usually by hiking or climbing

- Humanitarian and disaster response
  - Search and rescue workers—respondents to natural disasters such as earthquakes, fires, tsunamis, etc.
  - Health care workers responding to public health emergencies abroad
- Immigrants—persons who come to a country to take up permanent residence
- International adoption
- Last-minute traveler
- LGBTQ+ travelers
- Mass gathering tourist
- Medical needs—traveler with comorbidities (e.g., chronic illness, severe allergies, immunocompromised, disabilities)
- Medical and dental tourist—a person who seeks treatment or procedures abroad because of lower cost or lack of availability at home
- Migrants—a worker who moves from place to place to do seasonal work
- Missioners—travelers with a religious affiliation making a commitment of three months or more to live and work in a community, often one lacking resources
- Multi-generational travelers—trips that bring together several generations of a family
- Pilgrims-persons who travel to holy places or shrines for religious purposes
- Pleasure travelers
  - Vacationers—short-term or extended
  - Adventure or sports traveler—includes travelers who engage in high-risk activities:
    - Mountaineering
    - SCUBA diving
    - Spelunking
    - Open-water sailing races—team or solo
    - Long-distance motorcycling

- o Space travel
- o Triathlons
- Destination events—weddings, anniversaries, etc.
- "Babymooners"—couples taking a last vacation before childbirth
- Cruise travelers—persons traveling by ocean ships or river boats
- Pregnant and breastfeeding travelers—currently pregnant, trying to become pregnant
- Refugee—a person who has been forced to leave his or her country to escape war, persecution, or natural disasters
- Researchers—persons traveling for short or long durations to conduct research projects, including field research (e.g., anthropologists, archeologists, geologists, etc.)
- Remote travelers—persons seeking to go "off the grid" to regions without such services as mass communication, mass transit, translators, etc.
- Romance tourism—individuals traveling to meet persons encountered via the internet
- Seniors—persons over 60; often travel for a longer duration
- Sex tourism—persons who travel with the expectation of sexual encounters
- Unaccompanied minors—children under the legal age of majority who are traveling, often by plane or train, without a parent, guardian, or other responsible adult
- Vagabonds—travelers with no set itinerary; open-ended travel
- Voluntourism—when a traveler includes community service as part of a trip that may have a primary focus on tourism, business, or education
- VFR traveler—see below
- War zone traveler—tourist who chooses to travel to hostile regions

Vector-borne diseases. Illnesses caused by pathogens and parasites in human populations. (CDC)

Vectors. Organisms that transmit pathogens and parasites from one infected person (or animal) to another, causing serious diseases in human populations. (CDC)

VFR. VFRs are travelers born in a resource-poor region of the world, who now live in industrialized nations and return to their country of birth to visit friends and relatives; may also include first- and second-generation families returning to their birthplace; or travelers who seek brides. (CDC)

WHO. The World Health Organization, a United Nations agency headquartered in Geneva, is concerned with international public health. WHO publishes the International Health Regulations, which govern the reporting of certain infections by its member countries, including the United States. It also publishes travel health guidelines in its "Green Book" *International Travel and Health.* (https://www.who.int/ith/en/)

References

"ACIP Vaccine Administration Guidelines for Immunization," June 21, 2019. https://www.cdc.gov/vaccines/hcp/acip-recs/general-recs/administration.html.

American Society of Tropical Medicine & Hygiene (ASTMH). Accessed September 30, 2020. https://www.astmh.org/.

American Travel Health Nurses Association (ATHNA). Accessed September 30, 2020. https://www.athna.org/.

Angell, S. Y., and M. S. Cetron. "Health Disparities among Travelers Visiting Friends and Relatives Abroad." *Annals of Internal Medicine*, 142, no. 1 (January 4, 2005): 67–72.

Auerbach, Paul S., Tracy A. Cushing, and N. Stuart Harris. *Auerbach's Wilderness Medicine*. Philadelphia, PA: Elsevier, 2017.

The Australian Immunisation Handbook. *The Australian Immunisation Handbook*. The Australian Immunisation Handbook, September 14, 2018. https://immunisationhandbook.health.gov.au/.

Bacaner, N. "Travel Medicine Considerations for North American Immigrants Visiting Friends and Relatives." *JAMA: The Journal of the American Medical Association*, 291, no. 23 (June 16, 2004): 2856–64.

Bazaldua, Oralia V., and Jeri Sias. "Cultural Competence: A Pharmacy Perspective." *Journal of Pharmacy Practice*, 17, no. 3 (2004): 160–66. https://doi.org/10.1177/0897190004264812.

Bazemore, A. W. "The Pre-Travel Consultation." *American Family Physician*, 80(6), 80, no. 62009 (September 15, 2009): 583–90.

Benner, Patricia. "From Novice to Expert." The *American Journal of Nursing*, 82, no. 3 (March 1982): 402. https://doi.org/10.2307/3462928.

Bhadelia, Nahid, Mary Klotman, and Daniel Caplivski. "The HIV-Positive Traveler." *The American Journal of Medicine*, 120, no. 7 (July 2007): 574–80. https://doi.org/10.1016/j.amjmed.2007.02.018.

Bhatta, Prakash, Padam Simkhada, Edwin Van Teijlingen, and Susanna Maybin. "A Questionnaire Study of Voluntary Service Overseas (VSO) Volunteers: Health Risk and Problems Encountered." *Journal of Travel Medicine*, 16, no. 5 (2009): 332–37. https://doi.org/10.1111/j.1708-8305.2009.00342.x.

Brewer, Katie. "Scope and Standards-of-Practice Documents: Guiding You to Leadership Success." *American Nurse*, October 11, 2019. https://www.myamericannurse.com/scope-and-standards-of-practice-documents-guiding-you-to-leadership-success/.

Carroll, I. Dale, and Damian C. Williams. "Pre-Travel Vaccination and Medical Prophylaxis in the Pregnant Traveler." *Travel Medicine and Infectious Disease*, 6, no. 5 (September 2008): 259–75. https://doi.org/10.1016/j.tmaid.2008.04.005.

Chen, Lin H., Karin Leder, and Mary E. Wilson. "Business Travelers: Vaccination Considerations for This Population." *Expert Review of Vaccines,* 12, no. 4 (2013): 453–66. https://doi.org/10.1586/erv.13.16.

Chen, Lin H., Mary E. Wilson, Xiaohong Davis, Louis Loutan, Eli Schwartz, Jay Keystone, Devon Hale, et al. "Illness in Long-Term Travelers Visiting GeoSentinel Clinics." *Emerging Infectious Diseases,* 15, no. 11 (2009): 1773–82. https://doi.org/10.3201/eid1511.090945.

"Code of Ethics for Nurses with Interpretive Statements." Silver Springs: American Nurses Association, 2015.

"Cultural Competency in Baccalaureate Nursing Education." Washington, DC: American Association of Colleges of Nursing (AACN), 2008.

Doan, Sylvia, and Russell W. Steele. "Advice for Families Traveling to Developing Countries With Young Children." *Clinical Pediatrics,* 52, no. 9 (2013): 803–11. https://doi.org/10.1177/0009922813491313.

Duffy, Mary E. "A Critique of Cultural Education in Nursing." *Journal of Advanced Nursing,* 36, no. 4 (2001): 487–95. https://doi.org/10.1046/j.1365-2648.2001.02000.x.

Ezeanolue, E., K. Harriman, A. Kroger, and C. Pellegrini. "ACIP General Best Practice Guidelines for Immunization." Centers for Disease Control and Prevention. Centers for Disease Control and Prevention, April 20, 2017. https://www.cdc.gov/vaccines/hcp/acip-recs/general-recs/index.html.

Finnell, D. "Best Practices for Developing Specialty Nursing Scope and Standards of Practice." *The Online Journals of Nursing,* 20(2), 2015.

Freedman, D. "Malaria prevention in short-term travelers." *New England Journal of Medicine,* 359 (2008): 603–612.

Freedman, D. et al. "GeoSentinel Surveillance Network. Spectrum of disease and relation to place of exposure among ill returned travelers." *New England Journal of Medicine,* 354(2) (January 12, 2016): 119–30.

Freedman, D. O., Chen, L. H., Kozarsky, P. E. "Medical Considerations before International Travel." *New England Journal of Medicine,* 375(3) (July 21, 2016): 247–60.

Fukada, M. "Nursing Competency: Definition, Structure and Development." *Yonago Acta Medica,* 61(1) (March 2018): 1–7.

Gilbert, M. Jean., ed. *Principles and Recommended Standards for Cultural Competence Education of Health Care Professionals.* Woodland Hills, CA: The Endowment, 2003.

Giger, J. et al. "American Academy of Nursing Expert Panel Report: Developing cultural competence to eliminate health disparities in ethnic minorities and other vulnerable populations." *Journal of Transcultural Nursing,* 18(2) (2016): 95–102.

Harper, M. G., and Maloney, P. *Nursing professional development: Scope and standards of practice (3rd ed.).* Chicago, IL: Association for Nursing Professional Development, 2016.

"Heading Home Healthy - Helping Travelers Stay Healthy When They Are Returning Home to Visit Friends and Relatives." Home. Accessed September 27, 2020. https://www.headinghomehealthy.org/.

Heymann, D. ed. *Control of Communicable Diseases Manual.* 20th ed. APHA, 2014.

Hochberg, N. S. et al. "International travel by persons with medical comorbidities: Understanding risks and providing advice." *Mayo Clinic Proceedings,* 88(11) (2013): 1231–40.

Huey-Ming Tzeng. "Demand for nursing competencies: An exploratory study in Taiwan's hospital system." *Journal of Clinical Nursing,* 12 (2003): 509–518.

Immunization Action Coalition. Accessed September 26, 2020. http://www.immunize.org.

Infectious Disease Society of America. Accessed September 26, 2020. http://www.idsociety.org.

International Association for Medical Assistance to Travelers. Accessed September 26, 2020. http://www.iamat.org.

International Society of Travel Medicine. Accessed September 26, 2020. http://www.istm.org.

Jenks, N. "Travel health: safety and preparation strategies for clinicians." *The Nurse Practitioner,* 37(1) (January 19, 2012): 1–7.

Keystone, J. et al. eds. *Travel Medicine, 3rd ed.* Elsevier Science Health, 2018.

Kimberlin, David W., Michael T. Brady, Mary Anne Jackson, and Sarah S. Long. "Red Book: Report of the Committee on Infectious Diseases," 2018.

LaRocque, R. C., S. R. Rao, J. Lee, V. Ansdell, J. A. Yates, and B. S. Schwartz et al. "Global TravEpiNet: A National Consortium of Clinics Providing Care to International Travelers— Analysis of Demographic Characteristics, Travel Destinations, and Pretravel Healthcare of High-Risk U.S. International Travelers, 2009–2011." *Clinical Infectious Disease*, 4, no. 54 (February 15, 2012): 455–62.

Leder, K. "GeoSentinel Surveillance of Illness in Returned Travelers, 2007–2011." *Annuals of Internal Medicine*, 6, no. 158 (March 19, 2013).

Leder, K. "Illness in Travelers Visiting Friends and Relatives: A Review of the GeoSentinel Network." *Clinical Infectious Disease*, no. 43 (2006): 1185–93.

Lowe, J., and C. Archibald. "Cultural Diversity: The Intention of Nursing." *Nursing Forum*, 1, no. 44 (2009): 11–18.

Mahadevan, S. V., and M. C. Strehlow. "Preparing for International Travel and Global Medical Care." *Emergency Medical Clinics of North America*, 2, no. 35 (May 2017): 465–84.

Maloney, P. "Nursing Professional Development: Standards of Professional Practice." *Journal of Nurses in Professional Development*, 6, no. 32 (November 2016): 327–30.

Marshall, G. *The Vaccine Handbook: A Practical Guide for Clinicians.* 5th ed. Professional Communications, Inc, 2017.

Mikati, T. "International Travel Patterns and Travel Risks of Patients Diagnosed with Cancer." *Journal of Travel Medicine*, 2, no. 20 (March 2013): 71–77.

Miller, L. C. "International Adoption: Infectious Disease Issues." *Clinical Infectious Disease,* 40, no. 2 (2005): 286–93.

National Committee of Vital and Health Statistics Report: Eliminating health disparities: Strengthening data on race, ethnicity, language in the U.S. (2005).

Noble, Lorraine M., Adrienne Willcox, and Ronald H. Behrens. "Travel Clinic Consultation and Risk Assessment." *Infectious Disease Clinics of North America,* 26, no. 3 (2012): 575–93. https://doi.org/10.1016/j.idc.2012.05.007

Notarnicola, Ippolito et al. "Clinical Competence in Nursing: A Concept Analysis." *Prof Inferm.*, 69, no. 3 (2016): 174–81. https://doi.org/10.7429/pi.2016.693181.

Nursing Professional Development: Scope and Standards of Practice. Silver Spring, MD, MD: Nurses Books, 2010.

"Nursing: Scope and Standards of Practice (3rd Ed.)." American Nurses Association, 2015.

O'Connell, M. B. "Cultural Competence in Health Care and Its Implications for Pharmacy Part 1 Overview of Key Concepts in Multicultural Health Care." *Pharmacotherapy*, 7, no. 27 (2007): 1062–79.

Office of Minority Health. (2001), National standards for culturally and linguistically appropriate services in health care. https://minorityhealth.hhs.gov/assets/pdf/checked/finalreport.pdf.

Patel, R. "Travel Advice for the Immunocompromised Traveler: Prophylaxis, Vaccination, and Other Preventive Measures." *Clinical Risk Management*, no. 11 (2016): 217–28.

Plotkin, S. A. et al. *Vaccines*, 7th Ed. Elsevier, 2018.

Purnell, L., and B. Paulanka. *Transcultural Health Care: A Culturally Competent Approach*, 3rd Ed. 3rd ed. F.A. Davis, 2008.

Rosselot, Gail. "Travel Health Nursing." *AAOHN Journal,* 52, no. 1 (2004): 28–43. https://doi.org/10.1177/216507990405200110.

Royal College of Nursing. *Competencies: Travel Health Nursing: Career and Competence Development,* London: RCN, 2018. https://www.janechiodini.co.uk/about/publications/.

Sanford, Christopher A. "Urban Medicine." *The Travel and Tropical Medicine Manual,* 2017, 17–26. https://doi.org/10.1016/b978-0-323-37506-1.00002-7.

Sanford, C. et al. "The Pretravel Consultation." *American Family Physician,* 94, no. 8 (October 15, 2016): 620–27.

Schlagenhauf, P., F. Santos-O'connor, and P. Parola. "The Practice of Travel Medicine in Europe." *Clinical Microbiology and Infection,* 16, no. 3 (2010): 203–8. https://doi.org/10.1111/j.1469-0691.2009.03133.x.

Schlaudecker, J. D. et al. "Keeping Older Patients Healthy and Safe as They Travel." *Journal of Family Practice,* 62, no. 1 (January 2013): 16–23.

Schwartz, Brian S., Regina C. Larocque, and Edward T. Ryan. "Travel Medicine." *Annals of Internal Medicine,* 156, no. 11 (2012). https://doi.org/10.7326/0003-4819-156-11-201206050-01006.

Sias, J. J. "Cultural Competency." Essay. In *Pharmacotherapy Self-Assessment Program,* 5th ed. Kansas City, MO: American College of Clinical Pharmacy, 2004.

Strong, M. "Maintaining Clinical Competency Is Your Responsibility." *American Nurse Today,* 11, no. 7 (2016): 46–47.

"The Essentials of Doctoral Education for Advanced Nursing Practice." Washington, DC: American Association of Colleges of Nursing (AACN), 2006.

"The Essentials of Master's Education for Advanced Practice Nursing." Washington, DC: American Association of Colleges of Nursing (AACN), 1996.

"Tool Kit of Resources for Cultural Competent Education for Baccalaureate Nurses." Washington, DC: American Association of Colleges of Nursing (AACN), 2009.

"Tool Kit of Resources for Preparing a Culturally Competent Master's and Doctorally Prepared Nursing Workforce." Washington, DC: American Association of Colleges of Nursing (AACN), 2009.

Toovey, S. et al. "Special Infectious Disease Risks of Expatriates and Long-Term Travelers in Tropical Countries. Part 1: Malaria." *Journal of Travel Medicine,* 14, no. 1 (January 2007): 42–49.

"Travel Advice." World Health Organization. World Health Organization. Accessed September 26, 2020. https://www.who.int/travel-advice.

UK Travel Health Nursing Competencies—Royal College of Nursing, 2007. https://www.rcn.org.uk

U.S. Department of State. U.S. Department of State. Accessed September 25, 2020. http://www.travel.state.gov/.

"Vaccines and Immunizations." Centers for Disease Control and Prevention. Centers for Disease Control and Prevention, May 26, 2016. http://www.cdc.gov/vaccines.

"Vaccines and Immunizations." Centers for Disease Control and Prevention. Centers for Disease Control and Prevention, May 26, 2016. https://www.cdc.gov/vaccines/index.html.

Warren, J. I., and M. G. Harper. "Nursing Professional Development Role Delineation Study Presented at the ANPD Annual Convention July 2015," n.d.

Wilson, C. "Standards of Professional Performance for Nursing Professional Development." *Journal for Nurses in Staff Development,* 28, no. 1 (2012): 43–44. https://doi.org/10.1097/nnd.0b013e31824164e8.

"2020 Yellow Book Home." Centers for Disease Control and Prevention. Centers for Disease Control and Prevention. Accessed September 27, 2020. https://wwwnc.cdc.gov/travel/page/yellowbook-home.

Index

Aedes illnesses, 8
age, in travel health nursing, 5, 7, 26, 29, 30, 31, 45
agents, travel, 29
air cruiser, 97
air pollution, in travel health nursing, 24
air quality threats, 32
airline hazards, in travel health nursing, 8
alert(s), 96
  to illness syndromes, 15
  travel apps and, 40
allergies, in travel health nursing, 3, 7, 9
  ethical responsibility, 31
  prevention counseling, 27–28
altitude risk, 5, 7, 8, 9
altitude sickness, in travel-related health, 24, 25, 27
Amazon, 30
ambulatory care, in travel health nursing, 37
American Association of Nurse Practitioners (AANP), 18
American Association of Occupational Health Nurses (AAOHN), 18, 23, 35, 89
American College Health Association (ACHA), 18, 23, 35, 39, 89
American Nurses Association (ANA)
  ATHNA and, ii, vi–vii
  Code of Ethics for Nurses with Interpretive Statements, 4, 31, 33, 63
  defined, 89
  goal of, 39
  Nursing: Scope and Standards of Practice, 2, 4
  recognition of travel health nursing, 4, 20
  requirements, 4
  Travel Health Nursing: Scope and Standards of Practice, 2, 33
American Nurses Credentialing Center (ANCC), 19, 42
American Society of Tropical Medicine and Hygiene (ASTMH), 18, 20, 22
  CTropMed®, 20, 42
  defined, 89

growth and development through, 34
  reliable source, 23
American Travel Health Nurses Association (ATHNA), ii, vi, 1
  ANA recognition of travel health nursing, 4, 20
  Ask Us Anything, 38
  certification process, 20
  Code of Ethics for Travel Health Nurses, 63
  Courses and Conferences website, 18
  defined, 90
  expansion of, 42
  goal, 4
  growth and development through, 34
  historical perspective, 36–39
  memberships in, 18
  Model Core Curriculum Guide, 17, 18, 19, 21, 38, 42
  nursing conceptual framework, 31
  reliable source, 23
  research and scholarly inquiry, 35
  TravelBytes, 38
  Travel Health Nursing: Scope and Standards of Practice, 2–3, 4
  Travel Well Research Award, 38–39
  U.S. nursing schools, 18
  values of travel health nursing professionals, 36
analysis, in travel health nursing
  analytical skills, 11
  analytical thinking, 23
  competencies involving, 47–48, 74, 77, 80, 81, 82, 84, 88
  data, 1, 21, 30, 47–48, 77, 81, 82, 90
  risk, 7, 17, 24
animal contacts, 10
antimicrobial resistance, defined, 90
application, in travel health nursing, ii
  code of ethics provisions, 31–36
  authority, accountability, and responsibility, 33
  collaboration with other health professionals, 35–36
  commitment to patient, 32
  individual and collective effort, 34–35

nurse practices with compassion
and respect, 31–32
research and scholarly inquiry, 35
responsibility to promote health
and safety, 33–34
rights, health, and safety of patient,
32–33
values, articulation, 36
competencies involving, 46, 54, 57,
62, 65, 71, 72, 75, 77, 80
standards, 2
*Application of Code of Ethics Provisions by
Travel Health Nurses,* 4
applied science, in travel health nursing,
46
APRN. *see* advanced practice registered
nurses (APRN)
armed conflict regions, 97
arthritis, psoriatic, 7
Ask Us Anything, 38
asplenia, 7
assessment, in travel health nursing, 1,
24
advanced beginner travel health nurse,
21
competencies involving, 45–46, 47,
52, 54, 55, 60, 61, 65, 67, 70,
81, 82, 87
comprehensive health and safety risk,
5–6
defined, 90
multiple determinants of health, 4–5
post-travel encounters, 9, 17
pre-travel encounters, 6–7, 14–15, 17
self-assessment, 65, 70
Standards of Travel Health Nursing
Practice, 45–46
subjective and objective data, 5, 21,
30
assistive devices, 7
asthma, in travel health nursing, 9, 25
ASTMH. *see* American Society of
Tropical Medicine and Hygiene
(ASTMH)
asymptomatic conditions, screening for,
10
ATHNA. *see* American Travel Health
Nurses Association (ATHNA)

attention deficit hyperactivity disorder
(ADHD), 7
attitudes, in travel health nursing, 7, 45,
91
attributes, in travel health nursing, 25,
31–32
audit, in travel health nursing, 80, 84
authority(ies), in travel health nursing
code of ethics, 33
competencies involving, 46, 80
expert travel health nurse, 23
graduate-level prepared RN, 15
institutional and public health, 9
legal, 91
prescriptive, 9
school, 29
travel health nurse, 13, 33
autonomy, in travel health nursing,
31–32, 63, 73
avian influenza, 32, 33

B

babymooners, in travel health nursing, 7,
20, 99
Bacille Calmette–Guerin (BCG) vaccine,
24
backpackers, 97
barotrauma with diving, 24
barriers, in travel health nursing, 29–30,
33, 45, 56, 81
behavioral psychology, in travel health
nursing, 1, 5
behavioral science, in travel health
nursing, 46
beliefs, in travel health nursing
competencies involving, 45, 51, 52,
59, 63, 65, 66
spiritual, 31
benefits, in travel health nursing, 6, 26,
29
competencies involving, 49, 59, 61,
64, 71, 77, 85, 86
economic, 94
free member, 38
biases, in travel health nursing, 31, 32, 65
biostatistics, in travel health nursing, 46
bipolar disorder, 7

bleeding disorders, 7
blogs, 16
breastfeeding travelers, in travel health
nursing, 99
bucket list travelers, 7, 97
budget, in travel health nursing, 73
bush meat, 10
business, in travel health nursing
consultants to, 1, 14, 30
traveler, 28, 29, 32, 37, 40, 41, 97

C

call centers, tele-health, 13
care/caring, in travel health nursing; *see
also* nursing care
ambulatory care, 37
care centers, urgent, 14
competencies involving, 8, 49, 51, 54,
55, 57–58, 59, 61, 63, 64, 69,
70, 72, 73, 80, 82, 85
continuity of care, 49
coordination of, 8, 57–58
emergency, 15, 30
follow-up, 33
medical or dental, 7, 25
nursing, 2, 3, 6
plan of, 51–53, 54, 61, 72
post-travel, 9–10, 26
for post-trip health management, 8
providers, 1, 3, 13, 14, 22, 40, 47,
54, 69, 90
quality of, 2, 34–35, 36, 37, 73
self-care, 6, 8, 29, 30, 32
travel care, 96
CareerCenter, 38
CDC. *see* Centers for Disease Control and
Prevention (CDC)
centers, travel health, 1, 14
CDC, 4, 12
tele-health, 13
Centers for Disease Control and
Prevention (CDC)
assessment parameters by, 46
defined, 90
diverse travelers, 40
*Epidemiology and Prevention of Vaccine
Preventable Diseases,* 18

goal, 90
health, defined, 40–41
*Health Information for International
Travel,* 18
publications of, 4, 14, 24
research and scholarly inquiry, 35
standard for travel health prevention
services, 27
travel health guidelines, 34
trustworthy source, 23
Vaccine Information Statements, 65
Certificate of Travel Health (CTH®), 20,
42, 90
certification, in travel health nursing
ATHNA meeting, 39
competencies involving, 81
expert travel health nurse, 23
interdisciplinary, 22, 23
post-baccalaureate, 18, 38, 40, 42
U.S. nursing, 19–20, 42–43
Chagas disease, 10
character, in travel health nursing,
33–34
chemoprophylaxis, 20, 90
children, in travel health nursing, 13, 19,
27, 31
Chiodini, J., 3
cholera, 24, 27
chronic illness, in travel health nursing,
7, 9
civil unrest, in travel health nursing, 23
climate, in travel health nursing, 7
hazards, 8
risk, 5
clinical environments, in travel health
nursing, 3
clinical findings, in travel health nursing,
10, 48
clinical nurse specialists, in travel health
nursing, 15
clinical support, in travel health nursing,
47
Clinical Tropical Medicine and Travelers'
Health (CTropMed®), 20, 42
clinics, travel health, 11, 13, 14, 15
code of ethics, in travel health nursing
authority, accountability, and
responsibility, 33

collaboration with other health professionals, 35–36
commitment to patient, 32
compassion and respect, 31–32
individual and collective effort, 34–35
provisions, 31–36
research and scholarly inquiry, 35
responsibility to promote health and safety, 33–34
rights, health, and safety of patient, 32–33
values, articulation, 36
Code of Ethics for Nurses with Interpretive Statements (ANA), 4, 31, 33, 63
Code of Ethics for Travel Health Nurses (ATHNA), 63
cognitive assessment, in travel health nursing, 45
collaboration, in travel health nursing, ii, 15–16, 22
  ATHNA and, 38–39, 42
  colleagues for, 33–34
  competencies involving, 54, 56, 72
  defined, 90
  with other health professionals, 35–36
  on research endeavors, 35
  in settings, 33–34
  Standards of Professional Performance, 72
colleagues, in travel health nursing, 21, 33–34, 35
  competencies involving, 57, 63, 64, 66, 67, 69, 70, 71, 72, 73, 74, 77, 79, 84, 87
colleges, in travel health nursing, 3, 11, 13, 14
commitment, in travel health nursing, 37, 39
  code of ethics, 32
  competencies involving, 73, 75, 98
  expert travel health nurse, 23
  lifelong learning, 20, 73, 75
committees, in travel health nursing, 22
communications, in travel health nursing, 3, 9
  advanced beginner travel health nurse, 21
  through ATHNA, 36, 38

with CDC, state, and local health departments, 28
  competencies involving, 45, 55, 57, 60, 65, 66, 69–71, 72, 73, 75, 87
  language courses, 19
  mass, 99
  monthly Constant Contact, 38
  with nursing principals, 3
  open-access website for, 38
  pre-travel consultation and, 34
  Standards of Professional Performance for Travel Health Nursing, 69–71
  written and verbal, 17
communities, in travel health nursing, ii, 1, 5, 6
  assessment, 90
  campus, 89
  care of, 93
  commitment, 32
  competencies involving, 45, 46, 47, 49, 50, 54, 58, 61, 63, 66, 67, 70, 71, 77, 82, 85, 87
  free member benefit, 38
  health outcomes, improvement, 3
  health services for, 95
  IAMAT list, 14
  immigrant and refugee health services, 28
  LGBTQ+, 36
  policies and procedures, development, 13
  pre- and post-travel patients, 21
  spread, 8, 28
  through evidence-based practice, 90
  travel health nursing professional, 29
  travel-related illness and injury, 26
  travel risks on, 11
  well-being of, 36, 94
comorbidities, in travel health nursing, 9, 27, 98
compassion, in travel health nursing, 5, 31–32
competencies, in travel health nursing, 2
  advanced beginner travel health nurse, 21
  assessment, 45–46
  collaboration, 72

content, knowledge of, 8
patient, 9
prevention, critical importance of,
27–28
risk reduction, 25
self-care management, 8
time for, 34
country restrictions, in travel health
nursing, 7
courage, in travel-related health, 33
COVID-19, 10
crime, 5
critical thinking, in travel health nursing,
70–71
cruise traveler, 7
cultural assessment, in travel health
nursing, 45
cultural barrier, in travel health nursing,
45
cultural competence, in travel health
nursing, 54, 57, 91
cultural diversity, in travel health
nursing, 54, 65–68
culturally congruent practice, in travel
health nursing, 65–68
culture, in travel health nursing, 5, 31
competencies involving, 17, 45, 49,
51, 52, 54, 57, 59, 65–68, 69, 82
considerations, 16, 30
factors, 10
health, 28, 41
sociocultural abilities, 29, 65, 90
Standards of Professional Performance
for Travel Health Nursing, 65–68
transcultural considerations, 16
variations, 66
curriculum, travel health, 11, 16, 18
ATHNA Model Core Curriculum Guide,
19
competent travel health nurse, 22

D

dairy products, unpasteurized, 10
data, in travel health nursing
analysis, 1, 21, 30, 47–48, 77, 81,
82, 90
assessment, 45–48, 61

collection, 15, 45–46, 62, 77, 80
competencies involving, 45–48, 52,
54, 58, 61, 62, 63, 77, 80, 81, 82
comprehensive, 45–46
health and safety risk, 5
subjective and objective, 1, 5, 21, 30
trustworthy sources, 23
decision making, in travel health nursing
code of ethics, 33
competencies involving, 45, 63, 64,
65, 68, 74
informed, 64
shared, 45, 68
skills, 21, 22
decision process, in travel health nursing,
23–25
deep-vein thrombosis (DVT), in travel-
related health, 8, 24
degrees, in travel health nursing, 14, 16,
18, 19, 22, 23, 38, 39, 40, 42
demography, in travel health nursing, 46
demonstration, in travel health nursing,
21, 22, 23, 34
competencies involving, 65, 70, 73,
75, 78, 80, 86
self-care skills, 30
dengue, 8, 24
dental care, in travel health nursing, 7,
25
dental issues, in travel health nursing, 8
dental tourists, 7, 98
depression, 7
design, in travel health nursing, 11, 17
competencies involving, 52, 53, 55,
56, 60, 61, 67, 73, 77, 82, 86
designations, professional nursing, 14
development, in travel health nursing
competencies, 3
competencies involving, 47, 49, 50,
51–53, 55, 57, 59, 64, 67, 72,
74, 75, 76, 79, 80, 87
Model Core Curriculum Guide, 19
policies and procedures, 11, 13, 15,
16
professional, ii, 3, 19
professional nursing knowledge, 2
technologies, 35
through ASTMH and ATHNA, 34

health, 9, 22, 25
outcomes, 6
post-travel encounters, 9, 11, 16, 26
professional nursing performance, 2
professional practice evaluation, 84
referrals for, 8, 10
self-evaluation, 84
Standards of Travel Health Nursing
Practice, 61–62
evidence-based practice and research, in
travel health nursing, ii, 1, 2, 3, 5
ATHNA and, 39
communities through, 90
competencies involving, 46, 49, 54,
55, 59, 60, 68, 71, 77–78, 85
defined, 92
findings, 35
guidelines, 23, 36
health and safety information, 28, 40,
41
interventions, 1, 5, 32, 35, 54, 77
nursing assessments, 30
nursing plan, 5
personal safety measures, 32–33
principles, 46
publication of, 42
recommendations, 32, 34, 39
scientific, 49, 87
Standards of Professional Performance
for Travel Health Nursing, 77–79
expats, 7, 97
expectations, in travel health nursing, 34
expected outcomes, in travel health
nursing, 47, 49–50, 51, 61, 91
expert travel health nurse, 23
extreme sports, in travel health nursing, 7

F

faculty, in travel health nursing, 14
Faculty of Travel Medicine, 3–4, 18, 20,
22, 42
families, in travel health nursing, 2, 6,
11, 13, 19
assessment, 90
care of, 93
with children of all ages, 97–98
commitment, 32

competencies involving, 46, 66, 70
generations of, 98
health services for, 95
prevention counseling, 27
relocation, 97
travel health nursing professional, 29
VFRs, 100
febrile illness, in travel health nursing, 8
federal guidelines, in travel health
nursing, 33
feedback, in travel health nursing, 56,
59, 60, 84
female genital mutilation (FGM), 92, 97
fever, hemorrhagic, 32, 33
filariasis, 10
finances, in travel health nursing, 5, 19,
34
barrier, 45
estimate, 49
findings, in travel health nursing
audit, 84
clinical, 10, 48
diagnostic test, 51
educational, 75
evidence-based, 35
research, 71, 75, 77–79
fitness-to-travel examinations, defined, 91
flexpats, 7, 97
flu-like symptoms, 9–10
Flu Vaccine Finder, CDC, 14
flying phobias, 7
follow-up, in travel health nursing, 8, 10,
22, 25, 33, 61
food and water pathogens, 32
food and water precautions, 25
fresh water-related illnesses, in travel
health nursing, 5, 8, 10
friends, in travel health nursing, 32
frostbite, in travel-related health, 24
functional assessment, in travel health
nursing, 45
funding, of travel health services, 74

G

gender, in travel health nursing, 5, 31
Geneva, 100
geography, in travel health nursing, 17, 65

H

health and safety, of travelers, ii, 1, 4
  ATHNA, 36
  competencies involving, 49, 50, 57,
    59–60, 66, 71, 75
  of diverse travelers, 17
  domestic and international travelers, 5,
    31, 32–33
  education and, 25
  epidemiology, policies, and regulations,
    75
  guidelines, 16
  hazards, non-vaccine-preventable, 27
  information, evidence-based, 28, 40, 41
  ISTM, 93
  local and national stakeholders, 11
  measures, 6
  outcomes, 49, 50, 71, 82, 94
  policies and procedures, 13
  population-based, 50
  pre-travel encounters, 6, 7, 32–33
  promotion, 33–34, 59–60, 66
health and safety risk, in travel health
    nursing, 5, 11, 15, 33–34
  assessment of, 45
  competencies involving, 45, 47, 55
  diagnosis, 47
  domestic and international travel,
    32–33
  global epidemiology of, 17
  identification of, 55
  knowledge of, 20
  non-vaccine-preventable, 27
  prevention, 94
  research destinations for, 21
  of specific populations, 31
healthcare, in travel health nursing, 40,
    42, 80
  delivery system, 36, 70, 82, 83
  environment, 2
  interprofessional, 58
  issues, ii
  needs, 52
  personnel, 6
  plan, 57
  policy, 73
  practices, 54, 64, 85

  pre- and post-travel, 67, 92
  products in, 87
  professionals, 60
  quality, 34–35, 73
  regimens, 64
  research findings, 75
  services, 11, 57
  standards of, 17, 70
  team, 33, 52, 63
  workers, 85
healthcare providers, in travel health
    nursing, 8, 9, 13, 47, 54, 69, 76,
    90
health centers
  college, 13
  school, 13
health counseling, in travel health
    nursing, 6, 8
health departments, public, 13
health diplomacy, in travel health
    nursing, 35–36
health disparities, in travel health
    nursing, 35–36
Health Information for International Travel
    (CDC), 18
HealthMap Vaccine Finder, 14
health promotion, in travel health
    nursing, 1, 5, 21, 59–60
health record, in travel health nursing, 8
health status, in travel health nursing, 5,
    29, 31, 94
health teaching and health promotion, in
    travel health nursing, 59–60
heat stroke, in travel-related health, 24
hemorrhagic fever, 32, 33
hepatitis A, 27
high altitude travelers, 97
history, in travel health nursing, 10, 15
HIV patient, in travel health nursing, 20,
    27, 65
holistic data, in travel health nursing,
    45, 92
humanitarian organization, in travel
    health nursing, 14, 32
human rights, in travel health nursing,
    35–36
human trafficking, 36, 63
hypothermia, in travel-related health, 24

I

identification, in travel health nursing, 33, 36
  advanced beginner, 21
  barriers, 29, 45
  competencies involving, 45, 46, 47, 48, 49–50, 51, 52, 53, 54–56, 57, 60, 61, 67, 75, 77, 80, 81, 82, 83, 84, 85
  health and safety risks, 7, 11, 15, 24
  health care services, 11
  outcomes, 49–50
  potential public health emergencies, 28, 41
  self-identified, 37
  transmissible illness, 6
  travel-associated disorders, 20, 25
illnesses, in travel health nursing
  advanced, 16
  Aedes, 8
  altitude, 8, 9, 25, 27
  avoidance, 1, 21, 30
  CDC travel health guidelines, 34
  chronic, 7, 9, 25, 41, 98
  competencies involving, 46, 51, 82
  febrile, 8
  food- and water-borne, 5, 17
  fresh water-related, 5, 8, 10
  life-threatening, 10
  management, 7
  mental, 36
  by pathogens and parasites, 99
  Plasmodium falciparum malaria, 10
  post-travel, 32, 33
  prevention, 5, 17, 27, 28, 41, 93
  routine, 9, 25
  self-treatment, 95
  syndromes, alert to, 15
  transmissible, 6
  travel-related, 7, 11, 17, 20, 25, 26, 27
  vaccine considerations, 41
immigrants, in travel health nursing, 11, 17, 20, 32, 98
  care for, 13, 26
  compassion and respect, 31
  competencies involving, 65, 67

competent nurse, 22
examinations of, 15
health services, 28
participation in care, 26
prevention counseling, 28
proficient travel health nurse, 22–23
status as, 7, 31
immigration status, in travel health nursing, 31
Immunization Action Coalition (IAC), 23, 92
immunizations, in travel health nursing, 3, 6, 7, 8, 24, 27
immunosuppressed patients, in travel health nursing, 31
immunosuppressive conditions, in travel health nursing, 7
implementation, in travel health nursing
  APRN, 10
  competencies involving, 49, 51, 54–56, 57, 59, 73, 77, 78, 81, 82, 87, 88
  evidence-based nursing plan, 5, 49
  health and safety measures, 6
  policies, 34
  pre-travel encounters, 8
  Standards of Travel Health Nursing Practice, 54–56
  travel health consultations, 32
individuals, in travel health nursing, 2, 6, 7, 11, 13, 14
  ATHNA website, 19
  basic rights, 35
  commitment, 32
  compassion and respect, 31, 32
  competencies involving, 46, 49–50, 51, 60, 67, 70, 73, 82
  ethical environment, improvement, 34–35
  health needs of, 41
  planetary health, 40–41
  prevention plan, 15
  self-care, 29
  transgender, 28
  variety of disciplines, 35
infections, in travel health nursing, 13
  advanced courses in infectious disease, 19

health and safety, 40
infectious *vs.* non-infectious, 9, 26
post-travel encounters, 25, 26
respiratory, 8, 9
skin, 9
vector-borne, 8
Zika, 25
Infectious Disease Society of America
(IDSA), 4
influenza, in travel health nursing, 32,
33
informal groups, in travel health nursing,
37
information, in travel health nursing, 2,
24
assessment, 45–46
collection, 10, 81
competencies involving, 45–46, 48,
52, 55, 58, 59, 60, 63, 64, 69,
70, 71, 81, 87
contact, for infectious disease
specialists, 21
global health related, 27
on immunizations, 35
from national and international
sources, 30
on patient's characteristics and
behaviors, 29
regarding global epidemiology, 23
from reliable sources, 33, 34
safety and security, 3, 5, 28, 40, 41
informed consent, in travel health
nursing, 31–32, 33, 63, 64
informed decisions, in travel health
nursing, 23, 64
informed refusal, in travel health nursing,
64
injections, allergy, 3
injuries, in travel health nursing, 16, 33,
40
competencies involving, 51
epidemiology, 34
follow-up care for, 22
musculoskeletal, 9
post-travel encounters, 6, 11, 32
prevention, 19, 27, 28, 41, 93
RNs, 15
travel-related, 17, 20, 25, 26

inquiry, in travel health nursing, 35
insect precautions, 25
insect vector diseases, 32
institutional policies, in travel health
nursing, 9, 14, 15, 22, 25
institutional privacy, in travel health
nursing, 46
institutions, in travel health nursing, 13
insurance, travel health
coverage, 7, 25, 39
trip, 30
integration, in travel health nursing, 30,
35
competencies involving, 52, 53, 54,
58, 64, 70, 77–78, 85
principles of social justice, 36
integrity, in travel health nursing, 33–34,
36
interdisciplinary alternatives, in travel
health nursing, 20, 42
interdisciplinary certificates, in travel
health nursing, 22, 23, 90
interdisciplinary professional
organization, in travel health
nursing, 37
interdisciplinary sources, in travel health
nursing, 46
intergenerational tourists, 7
International Association for Medical
Assistance to Travellers (IAMAT),
14, 38, 92
*International Certificate of Vaccination or
Prophylaxis* (ICVP) card, 8, 92
international conference, in travel health
nursing, 14
International Health Regulations, 100
international health regulations (IHR),
41, 93
International Society of Travel Medicine
(ISTM), 14, 92, 93
Body of Knowledge, 18, 93
Certificate of Knowledge (CTH®), 20,
42
competent travel health nurse, 22
growth and development through,
34
interdisciplinary professional
organization, 37

poster, 39
publications of, 4
reliable source, 23
research and scholarly inquiry, 35
international travelers, in travel health
       nursing, 5, 6, 7
internet, 7, 17, 60, 95, 99
internet-based search engines, 7
interpersonal circumstance, in travel
       health nursing, 47
interprofessional team, in travel health
       nursing, 57, 58, 67, 70, 72, 74,
       85
interventions, in travel health nursing,
       10, 18
    competencies involving, 49, 51, 52,
       54, 55, 61, 62, 66, 77
    evidence-based, 1, 5, 32, 35, 54, 77
    risk reduction, 32
    scientific knowledge and tele-health
       technology, 30
in-transit encounters, in travel health
       nursing, 9, 93
isolation procedures, 10, 21
issues, in travel health nursing
    competencies involving, 47–48, 55,
       60, 63, 64, 66, 69, 75, 88
    cost containment, 40, 41
    dental, 8
    ethical, 63, 64
    global travel health, 22, 24
    healthcare, ii
    intransit travel encounter, 93
    medical, 8
    NGOs, 93
    physical and mental health, 7
ISTM. *see* International Society of Travel
       Medicine (ISTM)
itinerary(ies), in travel health nursing, 5,
       6, 7, 10
    competencies involving, 45, 46, 49,
       51, 54, 72
    complicated, 16, 26
    hazards, 20
    health and safety risks, 11, 15, 27,
       28, 31
    pre-travel and post-travel assessment,
       17

risk assessment, 31, 32
with special needs, 21
variety, 22

J

Japanese encephalitis vaccine, 24, 27
Jerusalem Syndrome, 9, 93
jet lag, in travel health nursing, 8, 24
job descriptions, in travel health nursing,
       2
Journal of Travel Medicine, 24
judgments, in travel health nursing, 32,
       75, 91, 92
justice, social, 36, 94

K

kindness, in travel health nursing, 64
knowledge, in travel health nursing, 1, 2,
       5, 16, 40
    advanced beginner travel health nurse,
       21
    ASTMH Certificate of Knowledge, 20,
       42
    competencies involving, 45, 46, 47,
       51, 54, 55, 60, 65, 71, 72, 74,
       75–76, 77, 78, 82, 87
    of counseling content, 8
    current immunology and vaccinology,
       24
    expert travel health nurse, 23
    federal guidelines and organizational
       policies, 33
    global travel health issues, 22, 24
    ISTM body of, 18, 19, 93
    ISTM Certificate of Knowledge,
       19–20, 42
    lack of, 39–40
    patient and environment, 30
    of RNs, 19
    scientific, 30
    in specialty, 17, 18
    state nurse practice acts, 34
    travel-related illness and injury, 26
    travel vaccines, 24, 27, 41
    U.S. nursing programs, 18, 19
Kumbh Mela, 93

L

laboratory results, in travel health nursing, 48

language, in travel health nursing, 8, 19, 31
  competencies involving, 49, 52, 59, 65, 66, 67, 69

laws, in travel health nursing, ii, 16, 41, 80, 81, 82, 87

leadership, in travel health nursing, 1, 13, 14, 16, 30, 34, 35
  competencies involving, 55, 58, 60, 64, 71, 72, 73–74, 82
  in national travel health groups, 16, 22, 23
  Standards of Professional Performance for Travel Health Nursing, 73–74

learning, in travel health nursing, 6
  competencies involving, 55, 59, 60, 65, 73, 75, 76, 78
  lifelong, commitment to, 20, 73, 75
  self-directed, 22

legal factor, in travel health nursing, 30

legal parameter, in travel health nursing, 63

legal system, in travel health nursing, 3

leptospirosis prophylaxis, 25

LGBTQ+ travelers, 7, 36, 65, 98

licensure, in travel health nursing, 14, 15, 89
  post-licensure educational options, 18
  as RNs or APRNs, 16
  state, requirements for, 19

lifelong learning, commitment to, 20

lifestyle, in travel health nursing, 59, 90

life-threatening illnesses, in travel health nursing, 10

literacy, in travel health nursing, 45, 65, 69, 70

literature, in travel health nursing
  competencies involving, 52, 77
  expert travel health nurse, 23

London School of Tropical Medicine and Hygiene, 18, 22

M

maintenance, in travel health nursing, 1, 2
  competence, 33–34, 89
  competencies involving, 46, 47, 63, 64, 70, 75, 76, 77, 81, 85, 87
  ethical environment, 34–35
  integrity of profession, 36
  post-licensure educational options, 18
  self-care, 29
  self-respect, 34
  social media presence, 16

malaria, in travel health nursing, 8, 9, 10, 24, 27, 32

management, in travel health nursing, 15, 19, 32
  competencies involving, 55, 70, 72, 76
  health problems, 9, 22, 25, 26, 29
  post-travel encounters, 25, 26
  rabies exposure, 33
  risk, 16, 37, 76
  self-care, 8
  travel-related injury/illness, 11
  tropical disease, 19
  vaccines, storage, 24

measles, 26

medical kit, travel, 8, 9

medical letters, 8

medical tourism, in travel health nursing, 65, 98

medicine, in travel health nursing
  competencies involving, 47, 76
  educational programs, 11, 13
  travel medicine, 18, 36, 37
  tropical, 1, 5, 34, 35
  veterinary, 35, 41

mental health, in travel health nursing, 36, 76
  consultation, 25
  issues, 7

messaging, electronic, 6

methods, in travel health nursing, 1, 17, 19, 29
  competencies involving, 46, 59, 62, 71
  of contraception, 36
  evidence-based, 30

teach-back, 5
transportation, 30
migraines, in travel health nursing, 27
migrants, in travel-related health, 20, 98
migration, in travel health nursing, 23
military personnel, 6, 7, 14, 29, 32, 38, 76, 97
minors, unaccompanied, 7
missioners, 7, 11, 32, 98
Model Core Curriculum Guide (ATHNA), 17, 18, 19, 21, 38, 42
moral distress, in travel-related health, 33
morality, in travel-related health, 33
morbidity, in travel health nursing, 26
mortality, in travel health nursing, 26
motion sickness, severe, 7
motivation, travel, 7
motor vehicle accidents, 8
mountaineering, 5
multidrug-resistant bacteria, 26
multi-generational travelers, 98
multispecialty practices, in travel health nursing, 13
musculoskeletal injuries, in travel health nursing, 9

N

national conference, in travel health nursing, 14
National Public Radio, 24
natural disasters, in travel health nursing, 30
natural science, in travel health nursing, 46
needs, in travel health nursing, 3, 25, 26, 30, 33, 34
  additional screenings, 28
  advanced beginners, 21
  APRNs, 10, 19
  assessment, 29
  competencies involving, 45, 46, 49, 52, 55, 56, 59, 60, 61, 67, 75, 85
  competent travel health nurse, 22
  of individuals and populations, 41
  language, 67
  learning, 59, 75
  malaria medication schedule, 8

medical letters, 8
novice nurses, 20–21
personal protective equipment, 10
pre-travel encounter, 8–9
proficient travel health nurse, 22
self-care, 29
skilled travel health nurses, 40, 41, 42
special, 7, 21, 22, 27
Netherlands, 4, 37
networking, in travel health nursing, 3
New England Journal of Medicine, 24
New York Nurses Network, 37
The New York Times, 24
non-government organizations (NGOs), 11, 14, 93
notices, travel health, 96
novice travel health nurse, 20–21
nursing, defined, 93
Nursing: Scope and Standards of Practice (ANA), 2, 4
nursing care, in travel health nursing, 2, 3, 6
nursing practice, in travel health nursing, ii
  authority, accountability, and responsibility, 33
  collaboration with other health professionals, 35–36
  commitment to patient, 32
  with compassion and respect, 31–32
  defined, 94
  individual and collective effort, 34–35
  research and scholarly inquiry, 35
  responsibility to promote health and safety, 33–34
  rights, health, and safety of patient, 32–33
  values, articulation, 36
nursing process, in travel health nursing
  defined, 94
  health and safety of travelers, 5
  skills, 1, 21, 30
nursing professionals, in travel health nursing, ii, 1, 30, 33; *see also* advanced practice registered nurses (APRN); graduate-level prepared travel health nurses; registered nurses (RNs)

nursing programs, US, 18–19
nursing specialty, scope of, 4, 5
nursing standards, in travel health
nursing, 3

O

obesity, in travel health nursing, 11
ob-gyn, in travel health nursing, 13
objective data, in travel health nursing, 1,
5, 21, 30
obligation, in travel health nursing, 33
occupational health units, 13
ocean sports, 5
older adults, in travel health nursing, 9,
31, 99
ongoing education, in travel health
nursing, 6
organizational environments, in travel
health nursing, 3
organizations, in travel health nursing, 1,
16; see also specific entries
competencies involving, 54, 55, 57,
67, 73, 74, 78, 79, 80, 81, 85
competent nurse, 22
environments, 3
NGOs, 11
policies, 33
religious and humanitarian, 14
WHO, see World Health Organization
(WHO)
orientation manuals, in travel health
nursing, 2
outbreaks, in travel health nursing, 5, 10,
11, 30
competencies involving, 51, 52
defined, 94
global, Travel Health Notices
regarding, 90
infectious, 32
travel health nurses, 34, 41
outcomes, in travel health nursing
defined, 94
health and safety of travelers, 49, 50,
71, 82, 94
identification, 47, 49–50, 51, 61,
91
improvement, 3

outcomes identification, in travel health
nursing
expected, 47, 49–50, 51, 61, 91
outpatient settings, in travel health
nursing, 2
clinics, 13
variety of, 6, 13

P

Pan American Health Organization
(PAHO), 23
panic attacks, 7
participation, in travel health nursing, 3,
6, 13
ASTMH, 18
care of immigrants and refugees, 26
competencies involving, 53, 54, 55,
56, 60, 61, 64, 65, 67, 72, 73,
75, 77, 78, 80, 81, 84, 87
expert travel health nurse, 23
immigrant and refugee health services,
28
pre- and post-travel care, 42
in professional organizations, 34
proficient travel health nurse, 22
quality assurance activities, 34
teach-back scenarios, 30
patient, in travel health nursing, 29–30,
36, 37, 39, 40
commitment to, 32
competencies involving, 70, 71, 77,
78
counseling, 9
education and advocacy, 33
immunosuppressed, 31
post-travel, 33
safety, 3, 25, 32–33
pediatrics, in travel health nursing, 13,
19, 27, 31
peer reviews, in travel health nursing, 2,
15, 23–24
competencies involving, 70, 72, 75,
77, 79, 84
performance(s), in travel health nursing
appraisals, 2
improvement, 3
standards, 3

personal growth, in travel health nursing, 33–34

personal protective equipment, in travel health nursing, 10, 21

personal protective measures (PPM), 10, 94

personal safety, in travel-related health, 20

pharmaceutical industries, 3, 5–6, 8, 34, 39, 66

pharmaceutical interventions, in travel health nursing, 8

pharmacies, in travel health nursing, 11, 13

pharmacology, in travel health nursing, 1, 5, 16, 19

phobias, flying, 7

physical abilities, in travel health nursing, 29, 30

physical and mental health issues, in travel health nursing, 7

physical assessment, in travel health nursing, 45

pilgrims, 98

planetary health, in travel health nursing, 28–29, 40–41, 94

planning, in travel health nursing
ATHNA, 18
competencies involving, 47, 49–50, 51–53, 54–56, 57, 59, 60, 61, 68, 69, 72, 73, 85–86
events, 5
follow-up care, 22, 33
national ATHNA meeting, 39
proficient travel health nurse, 22
risk reduction, 5, 15
Standards of Travel Health Nursing Practice, 51–53
trip, 11, 30, 31, 32, 39, 41

plan of care, in travel health nursing, 51–53, 54, 61, 72

Plasmodium falciparum, 10

pleasure travelers, 40, 98–99

policies, in travel health nursing, 2, 35, 36
advanced beginner travel health nurse, 21
agency, 21

code of ethics, 33, 35
competencies involving, 55, 60, 62, 64, 66, 67, 70, 73, 75, 78, 80, 81, 82, 84, 85, 88
competent travel health nurse, 22
cultural competence, 91
development, 11, 13, 15, 16
implementation, 34–35
institutional, 9, 14, 15, 22, 25
organizational, 33
pre-travel and post-travel, 9, 25
site prevention, 10

political factor, in travel health nursing, 30

pollution, in travel health nursing, 30

populations, in travel health nursing, 2
APRN role, 89
assessment, 90
authoritative statements, 96
care of, 93
commitment, 32
communication with, 19
competencies involving, 46, 47, 50, 53, 54, 55, 60, 63, 64, 65, 66, 67, 75
ecological model, 91
emergent diseases, 91
health and safety risks, 31
health services for, 95
immigrant and refugee health services, 28
pathogens and parasites in, 99
pre- and post-travel clinical encounters, 11
risk reduction measures, 20
safety measures, 6
sexual health, 28, 41
special, 27
United States, 89
vaccine administration, 17, 27
vulnerable, travel concerns of, 36

post-travel encounters, in travel health nursing, 9–10, 22, 94

preferences, in travel health nursing, 27
competencies involving, 45, 46, 51, 59, 65, 66, 69, 70
cultural, 65, 68
language, 59

responsibility to promote health and safety, 33–34
rights, health, and safety of patient, 32–33
values, articulation, 36
psoriatic arthritis, 7
psychiatric conditions, in travel health nursing, 7
psychological abilities, in travel health nursing, 30
psychosocial assessment, in travel health nursing, 45
psychosocial barrier, in travel health nursing, 45
public health departments, 13

Q

quality, in travel health nursing
air quality threats, 32
assurance, 15, 34
of care, 2, 34–35, 36, 37, 73
defined, 95
health, ii
improvement, 64, 95
quality of practice, in travel health nursing, 80–83
quarantine, 15

R

rabies, 8, 24, 25, 33
racism, in travel health nursing, 31
recommendations, in travel health nursing
competencies involving, 55, 60, 69, 78, 81, 84
evidence-based, 32, 34, 39
for follow-up, 25
for future screening, 10
personalized travel medical kit, 8
primary and secondary prevention measures, 11
for vaccine-preventable diseases, 6, 8
recommended vaccinations, 95
reef fish, 10
referrals, in travel health nursing, 8, 9, 10, 32
appropriate, 21, 25

competencies involving, 57, 82
for emergency care, 15
in-country/abroad, 33
professional, 33
reflective practice, in travel health nursing, 2
refugees, in travel health nursing, 11, 17, 20, 36, 99
care of, 13, 26
competencies involving, 65, 67
competent nurse, 22
ethical responsibility, 31
examinations of, 15
health services, 28
migration of, 23, 25
participation in care, 26
prevention counseling, 28
proficient travel health nurse, 22–23
status as, 7
regional conference, in travel health nursing, 14
registered nurses (RNs), travel health, ii
information, 2
knowledge and skills, 19
nursing process skills, 1
nursing professional, 30
scope of travel health nursing, 14–15
state licensure as, 16
regulations, in travel health nursing, ii, 15, 18, 32
competencies involving, 52, 63, 69, 73, 75, 80, 81, 82, 87
health and safety of travelers, 75
IHR, 41, 93
International Health Regulations, 100
scope of practice, 22
U.S. nursing, 20
regulatory agencies, in travel health nursing, ii, 33
relatives, in travel health nursing, 32
religious beliefs, in travel health nursing, 31
religious organization, in travel health nursing, 14
remote travelers, 7, 99
repellents, in travel health nursing, 8
reporting, in travel health nursing, 6, 9, 25, 26, 32, 33, 41, 81, 82

S

safaris, 13

safety, in travel health nursing, ii, 1, 2, 3, 4, 5; *see also* promote health and safety

  code of ethics, 32–33, 34–35

  competencies involving, 45, 47, 49, 50, 54, 55, 57, 59–60, 64, 66, 71, 72, 75, 80, 81, 82, 85–88

  concerns, 1, 21, 30

  guidelines, 16

  health and safety risk, *see* health and safety risk

  information, 40

  measures, 6, 10, 29

  personal, 20

  risks, 6–7, 20

  vaccine, 27, 41

SARS-CoV-2, 25

satisfaction, traveler, 49

schistosomiasis, 10

scholarly inquiry, in travel health nursing, 35

school authorities, travel health nursing care by, 6

school health centers, 13

scientific evidence, in travel health nursing, 49, 87

scientific knowledge, in travel health nursing, 30

scientific resources, in travel health nursing, 53

scope of nursing practice, in travel health nursing, 2, 95

scope of travel health nursing, 4–43

  administrative and educational roles, 11

  APRNs, 15–16

  certification, 19–20

  commitment to lifelong learning, 20

  competency, levels of, 20–23

  conceptual framework, 29–31

  continuing education, 18

  decision process, 23–25

  encounters, 6–10

  environment, 30

  future trends, 39–43

  graduate-level prepared travel health nurses, 15

  immigrant and refugee health services, 28

  need and significance, 25–29

  nursing professionals, 30

  objectives, 5–6

  patient, 29–30

  planetary health as critical priority, 28–29

  prevention counseling, critical importance of, 27–28

  process, 12

  professional nursing designations, 14

  registered nurses (RNs), 14–15

  services, national and global role, 28

  sites, 13–14

  specialized travel health nursing education, 16–17

  specialty practice, entry into, 17

  U.S. nursing programs, 18–19

screening, in travel health nursing

  for asymptomatic conditions, 10

  protocols for symptomatic/ asymptomatic post-travelers, 23

seasonal risk, in travel health nursing, 5, 7

security, in travel health nursing, 3, 5, 29

seizure disorder, in travel health nursing, 11

self, in travel health nursing, 33–34

self-assessment, in travel health nursing, 65, 70

self-care, in travel health nursing, 6, 8, 29, 30, 32

self-determination, in travel health nursing, 32, 63

self-efficacy, in travel health nursing, 30

self-evaluation, in travel-related health, 84

self-reflection, in travel health nursing, 75

self-respect, in travel health nursing, 33, 34

self-treatment, in travel-related health, 20, 95

seminars, for healthcare personnel, 6

seniors, in travel health nursing. *see* older adults

sensitivity, in travel health nursing, 5

services, in travel health nursing, 2, 26
  clinical, 13, 14, 15
  in clinical encounters, 6
  competencies involving, 52, 53, 55, 57, 59, 60, 62, 64, 66, 67, 73, 74, 78, 84, 85–86
  consultation, 11, 14
  global role of, 41
  health prevention, 27
  immigrant and refugee health, 28
  immunization, 3
  medical and safety, 5, 8
  national and global role, 28
  patient care, 14
  pre-travel, 3, 34, 40
  prevention, 39
  risk management, 37
  subscription database, 23
  tele-health, 13, 15–16, 30

settings, in travel health nursing, 33–34, 35
  clinical, 64
  college health, 3
  competencies involving, 59, 64, 73–74, 75
  cross-cultural, 91
  for-profit, 3, 39
  local practice, 23
  novice nurses, 21
  outpatient, 2, 6, 13
  RNs, 14–15
  variety of, 42, 59
  work, 34–35

sex tourism, in travel health nursing, 65, 99

sex tourists, 7

sexual assessment, in travel health nursing, 45

sexual behavior, in travel health nursing, 7

sexual orientation, in travel health nursing, 31

sexually transmitted infections (STIs), 5, 8

shortages, vaccine, 39

signs and symptoms, in travel health nursing, 8, 10

sites, travel health nursing practice, 9, 10, 13–14, 18, 19, 22, 25, 26, 38, 42

skills, in travel health nursing
  advanced beginner travel health nurse, 21
  analytical, 11
  communication, 17
  competencies involving, 46, 65, 67, 69, 70, 73, 74, 75
  counseling, 21
  decision-making, 21, 22
  in disease diagnosis, 16
  documentation, 20
  graduate-level prepared specialty nurse, 19, 92
  nursing process, 1, 21, 30
  professional, in travel health nursing, ii
  RNs, 19
  self-care, 30
  self-directed learning, 16
  in specialty, 17
  travel health nurses, 40
  U.S. nursing programs, 18, 19
  written and verbal communication, 17

skin infections, in travel health nursing, 9

social factor, in travel health nursing, 30

social justice, in travel-related health, 36

social media, 16, 35, 78

social science, in travel health nursing, 46

social systems, in travel health nursing, 46

social unrest, in travel health nursing, 5, 32

societies, in travel health nursing, 5, 16, 32, 35, 38, 73

socioeconomic status, in travel health nursing, 31, 59, 66

spa, 7

space traveler, 7

specialized travel health nursing education, 16–17

special needs, in travel health nursing, 7, 21, 22, 27

evidence-based practice and research, 77, 78
population-focused data, 46
traveler values and beliefs, 52
systematic circumstance, in travel health nursing, 47

T

teach-back method, 5
technology(ies), in travel health nursing
  advancing, 40
  communication, 9
  competencies involving, 51, 54, 59, 85
  developments, 35
  tele-health, 30
tele-health services, 6, 13, 15–16, 30, 85
temporal assessment, in travel health nursing, 45
temporal barrier, in travel health nursing, 45
temporal circumstance, in travel health nursing, 47
threats, in travel health nursing, 10, 23, 32, 87, 97
tick-borne encephalitis, 24
tour companies, 8, 11
tour managers, 6
tourists
  medical and dental, 7
  specialty, 7
training, in travel health nursing, 1, 2, 18, 19, 34
  advanced beginner travel health nurse, 21
  competencies involving, 65, 70
  lack of, 3, 39–40
  level of, 9, 25, 26
  in post-travel care, 10
  primary care staff, 23
  proficient travel health nurse, 23
  RNs, role, 15
  staff, 9, 10
  travel health nurse, 29, 30
transgender individuals, in travel health nursing, 28

transpersonal assessment, in travel health nursing, 45
transportation, in travel health nursing, 51
  accidents, 5
  modes of, 7, 30, 45
trauma, in travel health nursing, 9, 25
Travax, 96
travel advisories and alerts, 96
travel agents, in travel health nursing, 29
travel care, 96
TravelBytes, 38
travelers
  air cruiser, 97
  armed conflict regions, 97
  babymooners, 7, 20, 99
  backpackers, 97
  breastfeeding, 99
  bucket list, 7, 97
  business, 28, 29, 32, 37, 40, 41, 97
  cruise, 7
  defined, 97
  diversity of, 17, 25, 26, 29, 40
  domestic, 5, 6, 7
  ecotourists, 7, 97
  educational, 97
  FGM, 92, 97
  green, 7
  health and safety, *see* health and safety
  high altitude, 97
  high-risk, 92
  humanitarian and disaster response, 98
  immigrants, *see* immigrants
  international, 5, 6, 7
  LGBTQ+, 7, 36, 65, 98
  medical and dental tourist, 7, 65, 98
  medical needs, 98
  migrants, 20, 98
  missioners, 7, 11, 32, 98
  multi-generational, 98
  pilgrims, 98
  pleasure, 40, 98–99
  pregnant, 99
  refugees, *see* refugees
  remote, 7, 99
  researchers, 1, 7, 14, 19, 30, 32, 34, 99
  romance tourism, 65, 99

competent travel health nurse, 22
post-travel, 16, 17, 25
RNs, 15
tropical medicine, in travel health
    nursing, 1, 5
trust, in travel health nursing, 23, 72, 73
typhoid, 24, 27

U

unaccompanied minors, 99
undergraduate environment, in travel
    health nursing, 2, 16
uniformity, in travel health nursing, 2
unique attributes, in travel health
    nursing, 31–32
United Kingdom
    published work of travel health nurses,
        4
    RCN in, 3
United Nations World Tourism
        Organization (UNWTO), 26
United States
    certification in travel health nursing,
        19–20
    in diverse practice settings, 14–15
    nursing programs, 18–19
    outpatient settings in, 13
    registered nurse curriculum in, 16
    resources in, 59
    travel health clinics in, 11
    U.S. Travel Association (USTravel.org),
        26
    yellow fever vaccine in, 14
universities, in travel health nursing, 14,
    15, 34, 41
unpasteurized dairy products, 10
urinary tract infection (UTIs), 9

V

vaccinations and vaccines, in travel
    health nursing, 3, 5, 6, 20
    ACIP pre-travel, 16
    administration of, 8, 17, 24, 27, 33
    BCG, 24
    cholera, 24, 27
    competencies involving, 57, 59, 65,
        66, 80, 81

considerations, 41
    dengue, 24
    Ebola, 24
    Japanese encephalitis, 24, 27
    new travel, 27
    non-vaccine-preventable risks, 15
    pre-travel consultation, 25
    rabies, 24
    recommended, 95
    required, 95
    routine, 95
    safety, 27
    shortages, 39
    storage, 24
    tick-borne encephalitis, 24
    travel, 24, 27
    trials, 15
    typhoid, 24, 27
    unnecessary, recommendation, 34
    yellow fever, 8, 14, 24, 27, 80, 81
vaccinology, in travel health nursing, 17,
    18
vagabonds, 99
validation, in travel health nursing, 19,
    29, 47
values, in travel health nursing, 31
    competencies involving, 45, 49, 51,
        52, 59, 63, 65
    for diversity, 67
    nursing professionals, 36
variables, in travel health nursing, 10
vector-borne infections, 8, 99
vectors, defined, 99
verbal communication, in travel health
    nursing, 17
veterinary medicine, in travel health
    nursing, 35, 41, 76
viral hemorrhagic fever, 32
visa application, 8
Visiting Friends and Relatives (VFR)
    traveler, 7, 28, 31, 65, 67, 99,
        100
Visiting Nurse Associations (VNA), 14
volunteerism, in travel health nursing, 40
volunteers, 7
voluntourism, in travel health nursing,
    65, 99
voluntourists, 7

W

The Wall Street Journal, 24
war zone traveler, 7, 99
webinars, travel health, 18
Weekly Morbidity and Mortality Report
    (MMWR), 24
Wilderness Medicine Society (WMS), 18
workplace, in travel health nursing, ii,
    34, 35
World Health Organization (WHO)
    assessment parameters by, 46
    defined, 100
    guidelines, 16, 24

IHR, 41
    publications of, 4
    standard for travel health prevention
        services, 27
    trustworthy source, 23
worth, in travel health nursing, 31–32

Y

yellow fever, 8, 14, 24, 27, 80, 81

Z

Zika virus, 8, 13, 25, 26